OH
NO
SHE
DIDN'T

The **Top 100** Style Mistakes Women Make
and How to Avoid Them

CLINTON KELLY

GALLERY BOOKS

New York   London   Toronto   Sydney

GALLERY BOOKS
A Division of Simon & Schuster, Inc.
1230 Avenue of the Americas
New York, NY 10020

First Gallery Books hardcover edition October 2010

GALLERY BOOKS and colophon are trademarks of Simon & Schuster, Inc.

For information about special discounts for bulk purchases,
please contact Simon & Schuster Special Sales at 1-866-506-1949
or business@simonandschuster.com.

The Simon & Schuster Speakers Bureau
can bring authors to your live event.
For more information or to book an event contact
the Simon & Schuster Speakers Bureau at 1-866-248-3049
or visit our website at www.simonspeakers.com.

Designed by Jane Archer (www.psbella.com)
Creative Direction by Megan Lesser
Illustrations by Gant Powell
Photographs by Steve Giralt
Photographs on pages 19, 31, 44, 122, 175, 200 by Pasha Antonov
Line art by Clinton Kelly, Jane Archer, and Megan Lesser

Manufactured in the United States of America

1 3 5 7 9 10 8 6 4 2

Library of Congress Cataloging-in-Publication Data
Kelly, Clinton.
Oh no she didn't / by Clinton Kelly.
p. cm.
1. Clothing and dress. 2. Clothing and dress—Humor.
3. Fashion—Humor. I. Title.
TT507.K414 2010
746.9'20207—dc22
2010015759

ISBN 978-1-4391-6316-0
ISBN 978-1-4391-6936-0 (ebook)

THIS BOOK IS DEDICATED TO:

_____ *

You're a peach.

Clinton

*Write your name here so nobody steals your book!
 Plus, people will think you were my inspiration
 and be, like, so jealous.

contents

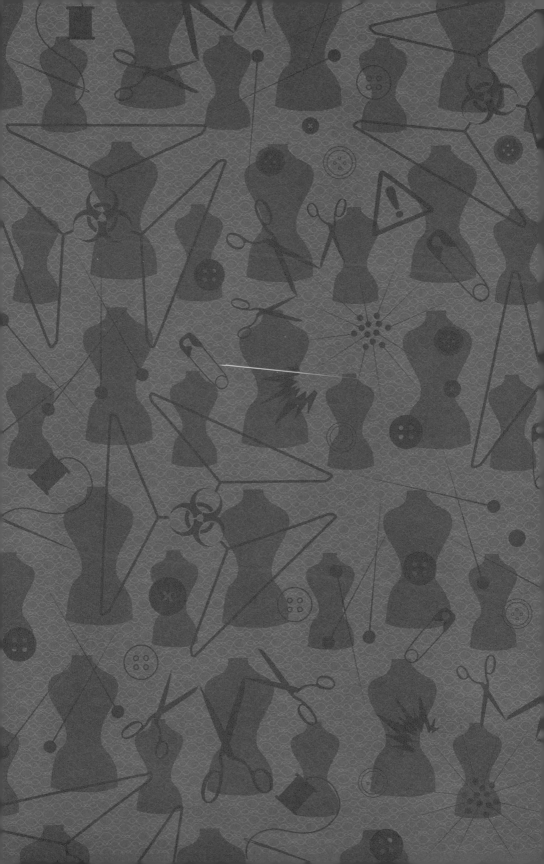

THE ATROCITIES I'VE SEEN...

I mean, seriously, sometimes I'm surprised I haven't already gouged out my own eyes. Truth be told, I did come pretty damn close once. I was in Pittsburgh, at the airport, or maybe it was Cincinnati. Doesn't matter, really. There I was, just minding my own business, reading the newspaper and waiting for my flight to board, when a couple of women approached me.

"Are you Clinton?" one of them asked.

This question always kind of bugs me. You *know* it's me. Just say hello and go back to your quadruple mocha latte. "Yep," I replied, and looked up to see two of the most horrific outfits imaginable. Both women—*both*—were wearing horizontal-striped turtlenecks tucked into high-waisted Mom Jeans with white cross-trainers.

"We love your show!" said one.

"We watch it all the time!" declared the other.

I smiled and said thank you, because I'm a gentleman. But inside my little head, I screamed to the heavens with all my might: *Why, God! Why do you hate me so much!*

Maybe I get a tad exasperated from time to time, but certainly you can understand why. I've spent the good part of a decade explaining, with as much patience as I could muster, why you shouldn't pair socks with sandals, why you might want to avoid tube tops after the age of forty, why elastic-waist pants are evil incarnate. But, evidently, not everyone is listening.

Still, I continue on with my mission to make America a more beautiful place. I'm like that Native American dude from the commercial who cries when he sees people litter. Except, I'm not crying. It's more like I'm laughing at you. In fact, he's laughing at you too. We're having gin and tonics right now, and I was just telling him that your outfit was revolting. And you know what he said?

"And how."

And how! Couldn't you just die? I almost peed my pants a little.

the mom jean

I was recently nursing a hangover on the couch and flip-ping through the TV channels, when I stumbled upon *The First Wives Club*. And after about a half hour of watching it, I realized two very important things. First, this is one of the worst movies ever made. I mean, seriously. The script is a steaming pile of pure poo. And second, Diane Keaton should stop shaking her head so much. She's going to give herself a goddamn concussion.

But I also noticed that Elizabeth Berkley's character (a mindless twit whose name I couldn't bother remembering) was wearing a pair of high-waisted, light-wash, tapered-leg jeans! That chick had a rockin' body and even *her* rump looked as wide and flat as a trash-can lid. It blows my mind. That movie was made in 19-freakin'-96 and women across North America are evidently still using it as a style guide.

Listen to me, ladies, and listen well; I'm only going to say this 27,352 more times before my career is over: Instead of the Mom Jean, go buy a pair of dark-wash trouser jeans. They should rest about an inch below the belly button. They should also hang from the widest part of the hip, straight down to the ground. Hem them so that they are about a quarter of an inch off the floor. Then, throw your old jeans into the biggest, most raging, blazing fire you can find.

Thank you.

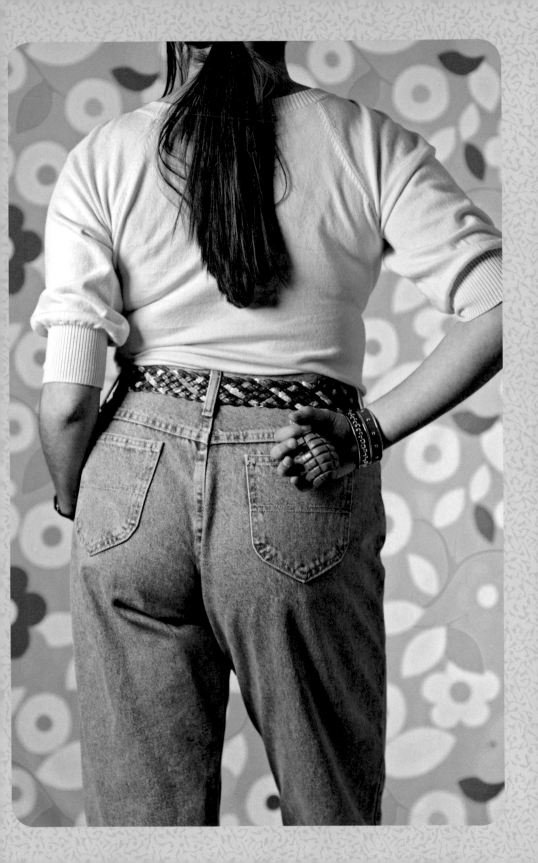

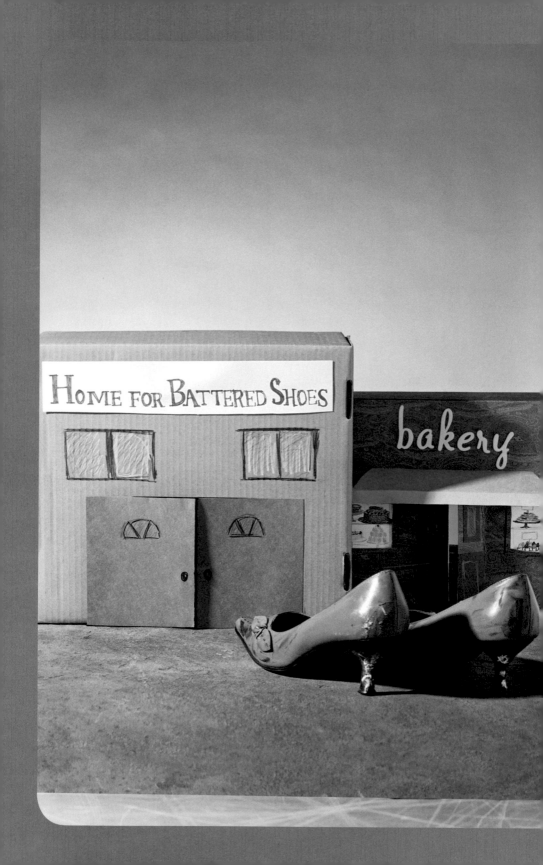

scuffed-up heels

Look, I don't know how much information your brain can accommodate, but I need you to clear out a little gray matter for the following concept:

The shoe always, always, ALWAYS sets the tone for an outfit.

Think about that for a minute. It's deep. It's the reason nuns don't wear stilettos and strippers don't wear orthopedic shoes.

You could be sporting a five-hundred-dollar haircut, flawless skin, an Italian silk blouse, a fierce Dolce&Gabbana pencil skirt, and a diamond the size of Rhode Island, but if you do it wearing chewed-up, gnarly heels, people will think you're a slacker. Seriously, I can't even tell you how many times I've seen women wearing shoes well past their expiration date, and there's this sloppy, careless vibe that clings to them. It's a little like, "I sleep on a mattress without sheets, I have Chinese food in my refrigerator that's older than Miley Cyrus, and the backseat of my car is filled with empty Big Gulps and ketchup packets."

Sometimes shoes can be repaired and sometimes they can't. The best way to find out is by visiting your friendly local cobbler. Mine's a peach! Going forward, if you know you're going to put a lot of mileage on a pair of shoes, bring them to the shoe repair shop *before* you wear them and ask for heel protectors or heel taps to be added. A very small investment of time and money will add months—maybe years—to the life of your shoes.

On a related note, I'm a big fan of the commuter shoe when executed properly. Your office shoes should be fabulous, but wearing exquisite crocodile pumps on the train, subway, and across five city blocks doesn't make a ton of sense. Buy yourself a shoe bag and carry your good shoes with you in a tote. Not only will the shoe bag protect the shoe, it will prevent contamination of the contents of your commuter tote. While you're traveling to work, wear something more comfortable—but still cute—like a ballet flat, a wedge, or a boot. You'll notice I did not suggest sneakers, and that's because they look really stupid with a skirt or a suit. And if you need evidence of that, it's time for you to watch *Working Girl* again.

fancy fingernails

I don't know when it became socially acceptable to airbrush your fingernails or apply rhinestones or paint each one with a different regular from *Dancing with the Stars*. I think it's a conspiracy among manicurists to destroy civilization as we know it.

There are two rules to chic fingernails: Keep them simple and don't let them grow too long. Really long fingernails are passé and creepy. And when it comes to color, keep them solid. If you work in a corporate environment, go subtle, maybe taupe or champagne. Or just get a simple buff job, which is always classic and clean. If you work in a creative environment—or don't work at all—you can go with a bolder color, like Chanel's Vendetta. (It's aubergine and fabulous.)

Are red nails okay? Yes, but you need pretty hands to pull them off or you'll look like a gargoyle.

What about French manicures? Well, they're about as French as that neon-orange Wish-bone dressing my aunt Kay used to pour on a head of iceberg lettuce. Plus, they seem to be the preferred nail style among the women who work at the Hustler Club in New York (so I've heard). There-fore, I cannot in good conscience recommend a *manucure française*. But the more I think of it, the more I like the idea of Maks on my pinkie.

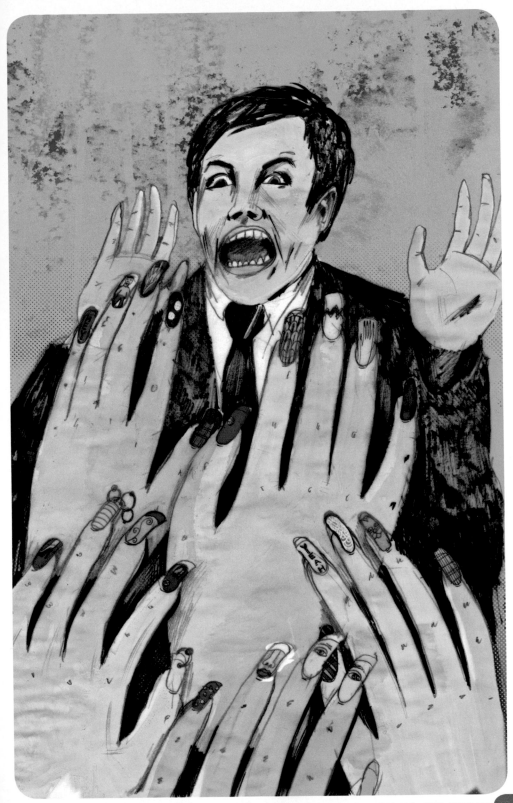

$$\begin{array}{r} 2\ old \\ +\ 2\ be \\ \hline \end{array}$$

wearing that crap.

Meet me in the parking lot after school.

 ♡ ← Mr. Kelly

catholic schoolgirl

This just in! Doctors at a very reputable university hospital have recently announced that any woman who has success-fully emerged from puberty and still thinks it's cute to be seen in public sporting a plaid skirt, a white button-front blouse, and knee-highs suffers from severe brain damage.

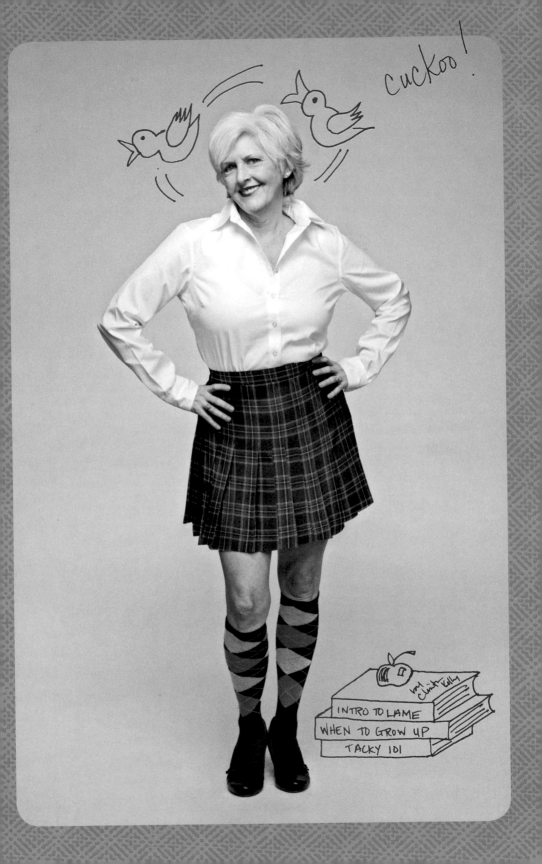

cuckoo!

by Clinton Kelly

INTRO TO LAME
WHEN TO GROW UP
TACKY 101

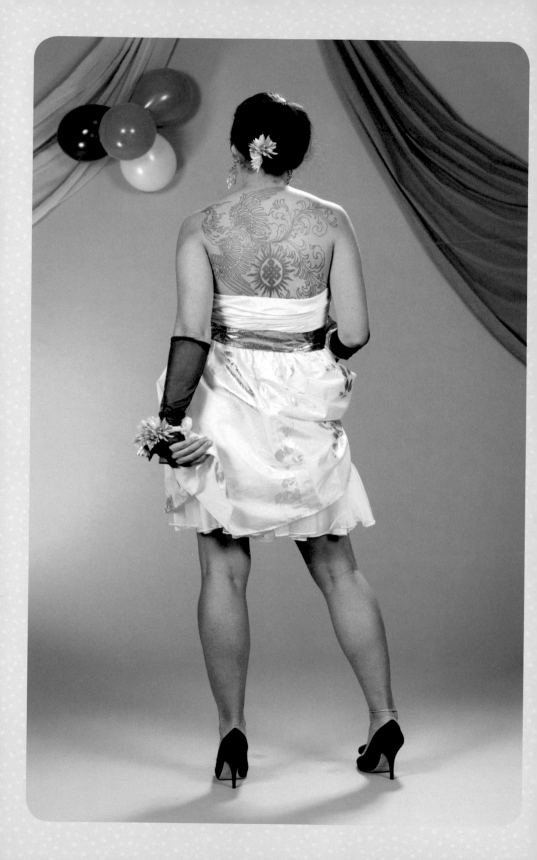

tattoos and evening wear

I went to this wedding once where the bride's mother had a tattoo of a teddy bear on her chest. How do I know this? Because she was wearing a strapless dress and it looked like the teddy bear was peeking over the top of the bodice. Every time I looked at her, I thought: *That lady looks ridiculous.* And the more gin and tonics I drank, the more it was like that damn teddy bear was taunting me. *Ha-ha, Clinton! This couple will be divorced in six months and you just gave them 200 bucks. Sucker. My name's Teddy. Wanna play?*

I know tattoos are really popular right now. And I'm pretty sure we're going to have an entire generation of old ladies and gentlemen who look pretty ridiculous with their wrinkled, inked skin under the hot Florida sun. But in the meantime, you should really think about how your tattoos relate to the clothes you're wearing. Let's say you've got a daisy tat on your ankle. Why would you wear a shoe with an ankle strap that cuts across it? That doesn't make any sense. Decide either to show the entire tattoo or to cover the entire tattoo. Now that you've got one, you have to work around it.

Quite frankly, if you're attending a formal event and you're *not* a rock star, I think you should cover up your tattoos completely, either with clothing or with a concealing makeup like Dermablend. It's the tasteful thing to do. And, Teddy, stop calling me.

Little-known fact:

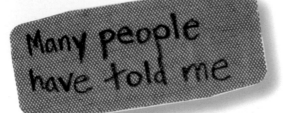

Many people have told me

I should be a foot model.

And by "many," I mean "three."

---

gnarly feet

You've got three corns, a bunion, a fungal infection, and a big toe that's got more hair on it than Matt Lauer's head. Please tell me, why are you wearing a strappy sandal?

Do yourself a favor and call a podiatrist. Until then, do the rest of us a favor and wear a closed-toe shoe.

Gross.

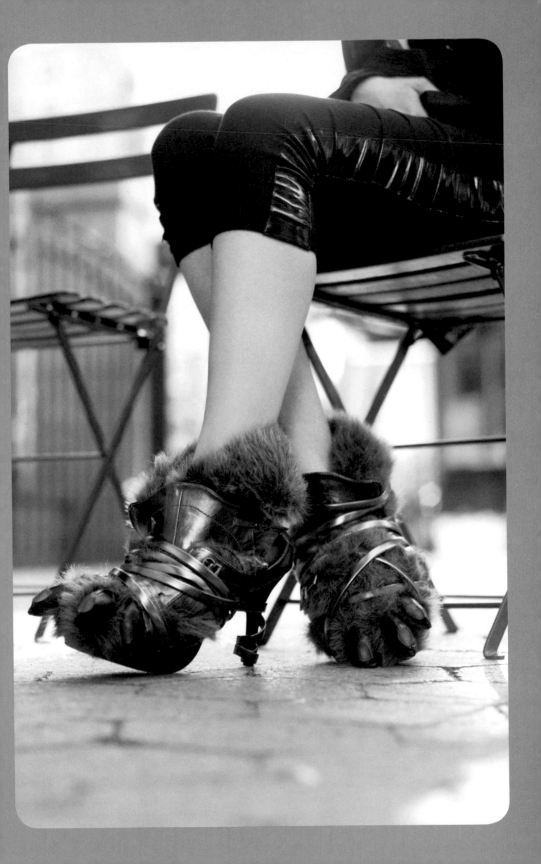

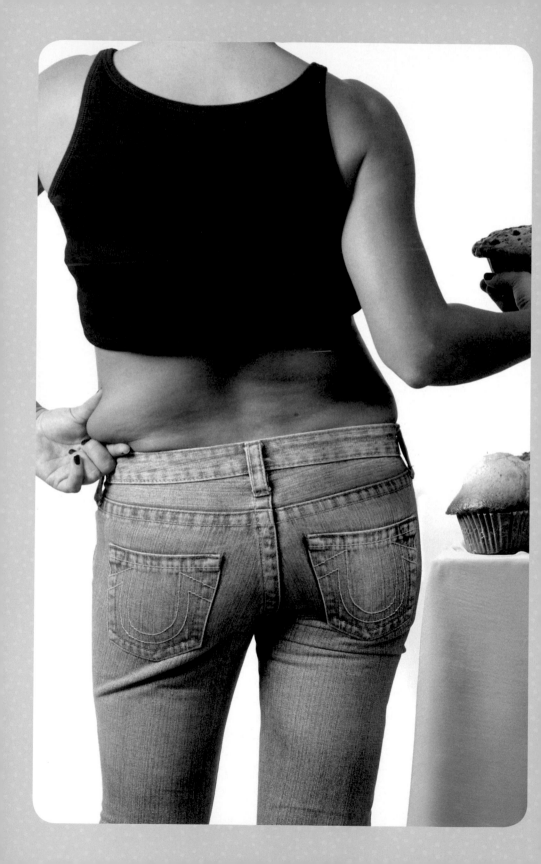

muffin top

Muffin top is one of those terms I'd be happy not to hear again for the rest of my life. God, I'm just so over it. Let's forgo the euphemisms and call it what it really is: a roll of fat hanging over the top of your pants.

I am going to digress now, because this is my book and I can do whatever the hell I want. Did you ever see that episode of *Murphy Brown* where Corky Sherwood explains how to tell if a man is gay? She says, "Tell him he has something stuck to the bottom of his shoe. If he picks up his foot in front of him to check the sole, he's straight. If he kicks it up behind him, he's gay."

Well, I have a similar test. Unless a man is in perfect— and I mean perfect—shape, he carries some amount of fat in his lower back; not in the middle, but right above and behind his hip bones. If you're vibing on a guy you just met at a bar, or at a Prada sample sale, casually touch him right on that fatty part. If he's straight, he'll do nothing. But if he's gay he'll flinch, wince, or jump like Liza Minnelli just poked him with a cattle prod.

End of digression. Someday you'll thank me for that tip.

If you want to avoid the muffin top, you have to keep the muffin in the pan! For most women, that means wearing pants with a slightly higher rise. If you carry *some* weight in the lower belly, a waistband that rests about an inch below your navel should be enough to prevent overflow.

But if you carry the *bulk* of your weight in your midsection, you'll probably need a pant with a waistband closer to your belly button to contain the squishy stuff. Or you can try tummy-taming shapewear, which should smooth everything out and hold it in place.

I should warn you: If you carry your weight in your midsection and need a higher-rise pant to control your tummy, you have to be extremely careful about tucking in your shirt, because it will only bring more attention to your midsection (see Tucking, page 159). And you should also be really careful about loaning Liza Minnelli your cattle prod. I learned that the hard way.

tracksuits

Is your tracksuit cool? Are you sure? Take this quiz and find out!

You are wearing a tracksuit at this very moment and . . .

You are J.Lo. *(Add 10 points.)*

You are in the Mob. *(Add 10 points.)*

You are fitness-walking in the mall and you are over the age of sixty-five. *(Add 3 points.)*

The tracksuit is velour. *(Subtract 2 points.)*

The tracksuit is vinyl. *(Subtract 2 points.)*

The tracksuit is pink velour with a word on the ass and you are older than seventeen. *(Subtract 375 points.)*

SCORING

0 to 23 points. Your tracksuit is acceptable. Congratulations!

-2 to 0 points. Here's the thing about tracksuits: If they're made of nylon, you obviously think you're living in a different decade. If they're velour, you've been brainwashed into thinking this is an acceptable casual look for women. I can pretty much guarantee that the manufacturers of such tracksuits are laughing at you—all the way to the bank. (I'll give girls under the age of seventeen a little leeway here because you're not old enough to know you're being brainwashed.) In general, if you're not in the actual process of working out, tracksuits make you look lazy, out of touch, or like some wannabe pop star. Try upgrading to jeans and a casual jacket.

Less than -2 points. You lose.

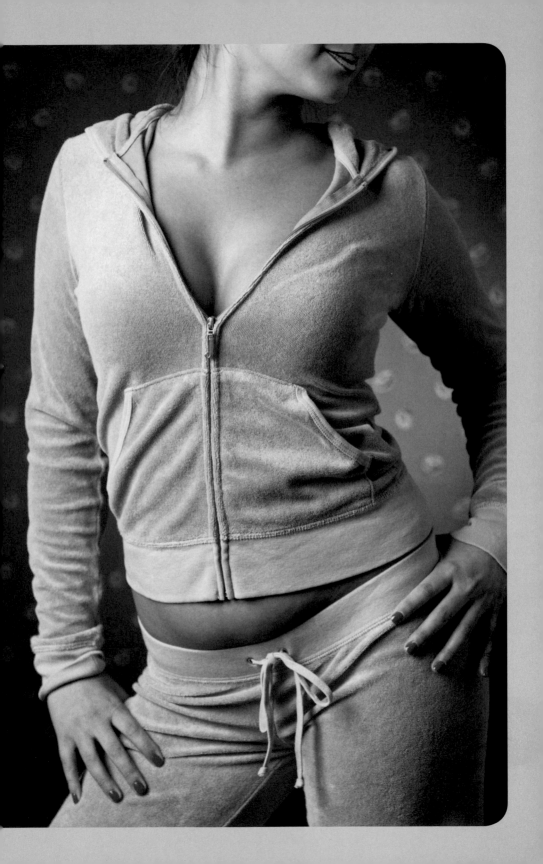

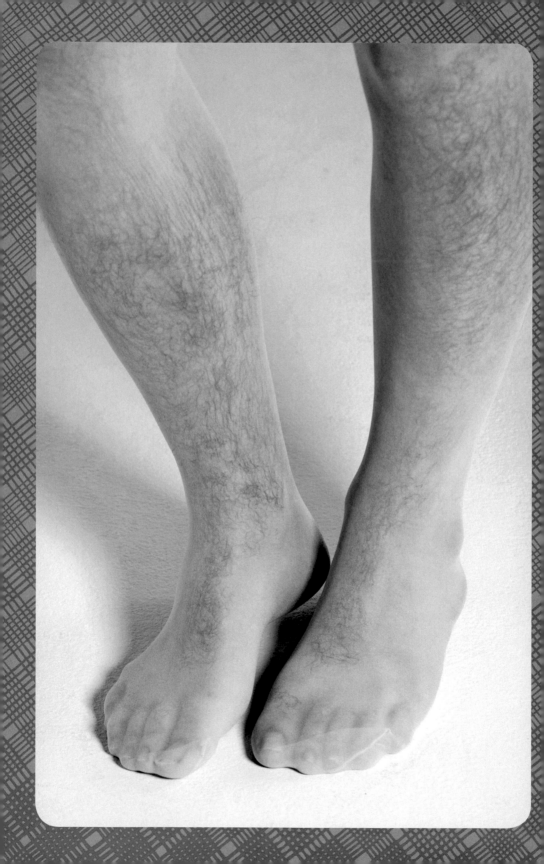

hairy legs under hose

Let me begin by stating that I strongly support a woman's right not to shave any part of her body if she so chooses; however, exercising that right should qualify you for mandatory military service. But that's beside the point.

For the love of all things holy, if you have not shaved your legs in a month, do not, under any circumstances, wear sheer hose! There are few things in the world as revolting as the sight of what appear to be a thousand tapeworms squished between a woman's legs and her stockings. Go opaque or go home. Better yet, use some kind of depilatory! And I hope all you drag queens and trannies out there are paying attention. Man up, and shave those damn gams. You too, Mo'Nique.

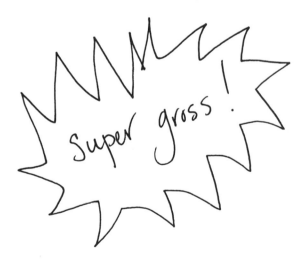

counterfeit anything

Manufacturing counterfeit products is unconscionable, because it's stealing and it's illegal. People who sell these fakes make me angry, and people who buy them have my sympathy. Yes, sympathy.

If you think that carrying a fake designer bag is going to make you more fabulous, your priorities are incredibly screwed up. That ill-applied label only tells the world you're ashamed of yourself for not being able to afford the real thing. If you can't afford an Hermès bag, who the hell cares? There are plenty of gorgeous, reasonably priced bags in the world, just waiting to be bought and carried with pride and style.

Sure, it sucks when someone else has the money to buy what you want, whether it's a bag or a car or a house or a swimming pool or a trophy husband. But that doesn't give you the right to steal profits from Hermès or Gucci or Prada or even Kate Spade.

Just be the best, most authentic version of you!

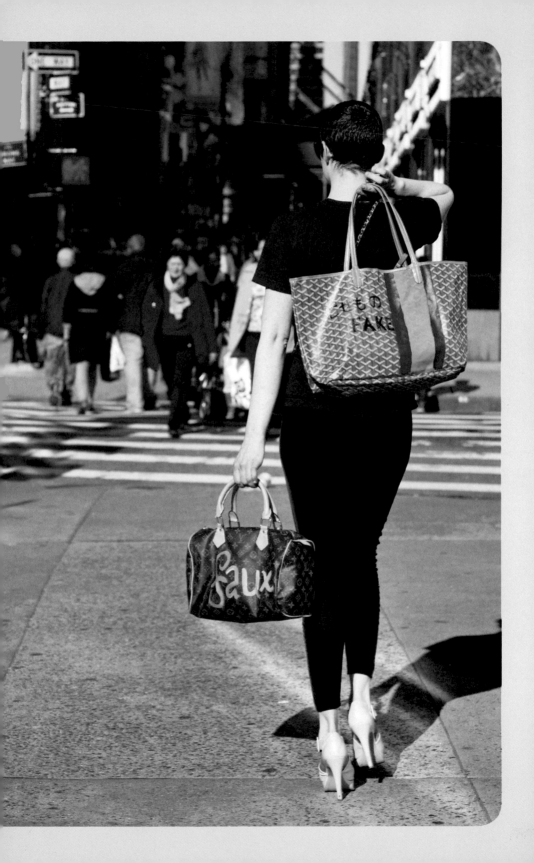

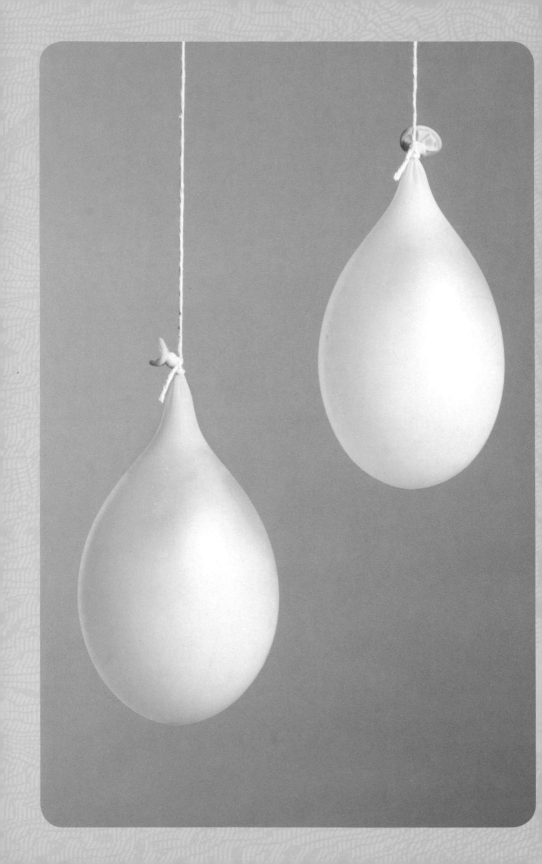

low boobies

Wherever your boobs rest naturally is just fine, and I hope you love them.

I will tell you, however, that pendulous breasts don't look so good in clothes and that's because clothes aren't constructed to accommodate a bust that hits the belly button. Clothes are designed on dress forms. Where is the bust on a dress form? About halfway between the shoulder and the elbow. (I know dress forms don't have elbows, smarty-pants. Try to imagine where the elbow would be.)

boobs go here →

So, if you want clothes to fit you better, it would behoove you to hoist your boobies up to that general position. You could have a doctor do that for you. *Or* you could try an absolutely incredible new product! It's called . . . a good bra.

How do you get a good bra? You go to a professional bra fitter, not the sixteen-year-old who works at a lingerie shop in the mall after school.

Most women I've worked with discover after a professional bra fitting that they are smaller in the band and bigger in the cup than they had thought. This is usually a welcome discovery, because if a bra fits better under the bust, the band can do the vast majority of the bra's work, rather than the straps. This will result in a more comfortable fit. If your bra is sliding down your rib cage, even just a little, the straps are forced to hold up the boobs. That means they'll be more likely to dig into your shoulders and cause fatigue.

Even when you know your bra size, you should try on a bra in a store before you buy it—especially if you're buying a different brand. There's no government office that regulates bra fit, so a 36DD in one brand or style might fit you, while a 34DDD in another might be the best choice.

Please, please, please . . . for the sake of fit and silhouette, give the girls a lift! They could use a little pick-me-up, and so could you:

1...2...3...4... Get your boobies off the floor!
5... 6... 7... 8... Now's the time to elevate!

applying makeup in public

Truly chic women have an air of mystery about them. They create and maintain the illusion that they roll out of bed looking perfect, even if their appearance is more engineered than a Dubai skyscraper.

Ladies, don't divulge your beauty secrets—any of them. Beautiful people have their blackheads squeezed, their colons irrigated, and their ear wax candled. But they don't let any Tom, Dick, or Harry watch. The same rule applies to curling your eyelashes while you're on the bus, applying lipstick at the dinner table, or powdering your forehead in the lunchroom. It's gross. It's rude. And it's beneath you. They put mirrors in bathrooms for a reason—use them.

P.S. If I look in my rearview mirror and see you applying makeup while driving your car at 60 m.p.h., I will intentionally slam on my brakes. So watch yourself, sister

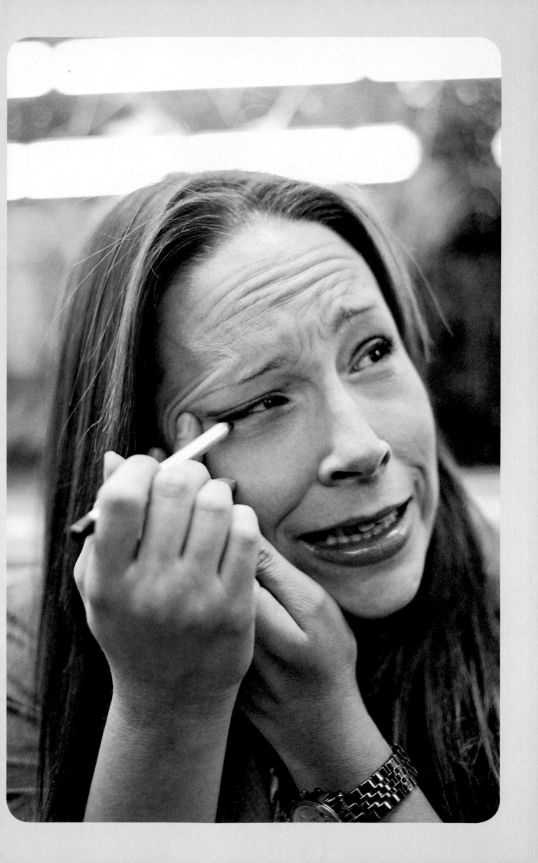

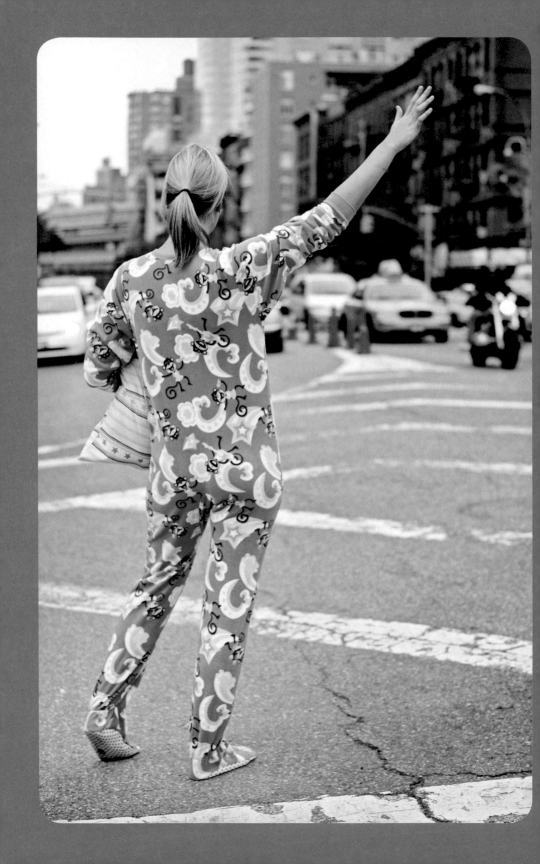

pajamas in public

I have a fantasy that I'd like to share with you. I've written it as a short screenplay. I play the MAN ON LOUDSPEAKER.

SETTING

A suburban supermarket. Young, pretty moms are pushing grocery carts. Muscular stock boys are straightening the shelves of canned tomatoes and diapers. Muzak plays in the background—"Groove Is in the Heart" by Deee-lite. A thirtysomething woman strolls in wearing an oversize Mickey Mouse sweatshirt and flannel pajama bottoms. Oblivious to the disapproving looks she is receiving, the woman lumbers to the frozen food section. As she contemplates ice cream flavors, an announcement is made over the PA system.

MAN ON LOUDSPEAKER

"Pardon the interruption, ladies and gentlemen, but can a store employee please report to aisle five to clean up a broken jar of pickles. I repeat. Clean up in aisle five. Oh, and while I have your attention, there is a hot mess in the freezer section too. Yes, lady in pajamas, I'm talking to you. I think I speak on behalf of everyone here today when I say that you look like a lazy sack of shit. We all got dressed this morning, but evidently you can't manage the most simple of human tasks: putting on pants. Please put the ice cream down and leave. You may return once you put on actual clothes."

The other customers and employees cheer. The woman runs out of the store, hanging her head in shame. Someone throws a handful of pistachios at her, but they mostly miss.

The End.

If anyone knows the temptation of spending a day at home in pajamas, it is I. In fact, I wrote most of this book while wearing pajamas. They're cashmere, but that's not important right now. More important, pajamas should not leave the house! Is it appropriate to wear a ball gown to work? Is it appropriate to wear a bikini to a PTA meeting? Is it appropriate to attend an animal rights rally in a mink coat? No, no, and no! So don't be an idiot.

If you've got errands to run, throw on some jeans, a blouse, and a cute flat, boot, or sandal. And maybe people will stop calling you a pathetic slob behind your back.

colored suits

I'd like to use this page to apologize to my sister, Jodi, whom I took shopping in the early 1990s. She needed an interview suit for her first job. I don't know if it was a lapse in judgment on my part, or a small undiagnosed brain aneurism, but I convinced her to buy a skirt suit in a shade of Concord grape with a seven-button jacket. Good God. If only she had applied for a job as a flight attendant for Smucker's Air, she would have been golden.

Colored suits might go in and out of style, but neutral suits don't. Madam Secretary of State: Are you reading this? A black, gray, navy, brown, or khaki suit will give you a lot more mileage, especially in a classic cut. Classic, meaning one, two, or three buttons, without a lot of tricky details, and of course fit is everything. Then add color, texture, pattern, and shine with your underpinning and accessories. (See All Solids All the Time, page 166.)

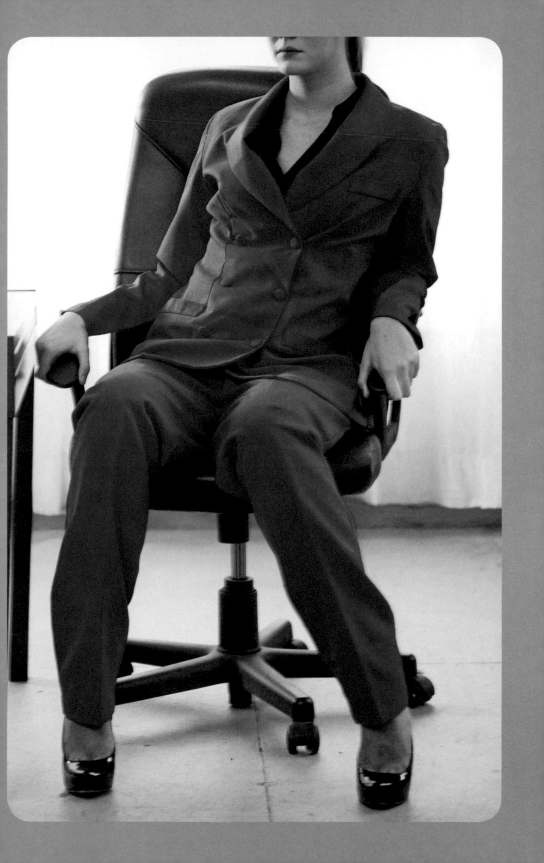

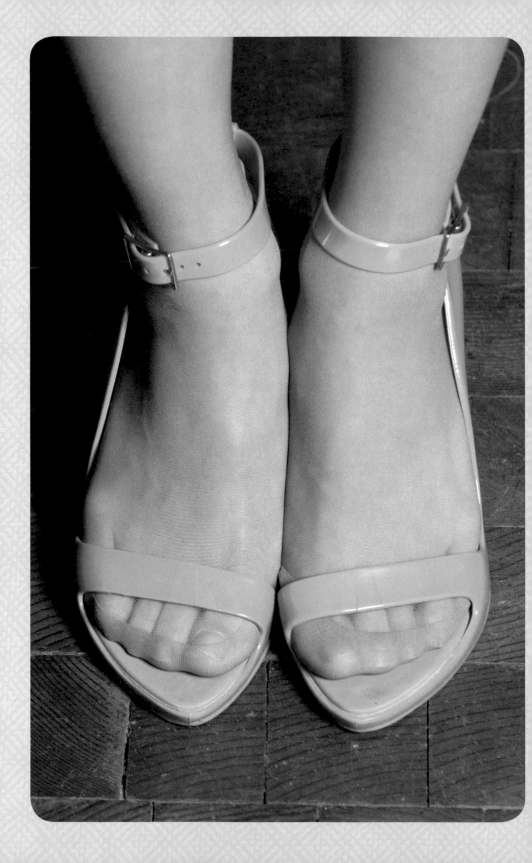

reinforced toe

I wish I didn't have to devote a split second of my life stating something as obvious as this: Don't wear reinforced-toe hose with open-toe shoes. But I do. Such is my lot in life and I've decided to be Zen with it. And by "Zen with," I mean "bitter about."

Can you wear seamless hose with open-toe shoes? Sure, knock yourself out. But those open-toe shoes had better not be slingbacks, sandals, or mules, because you'll look like an ass. Remember: No heel, no hose.

tramp stamps at work

There are certain occasions when flashing your lower-back tattoo is completely appropriate, and maybe even sexy depending on one's taste: at "the club" or at "the strip club" or during a reverse cowgirl. Not so chic, however, is when you bend over to pick up your dropped pen during a sales presentation and that thing is all up in the CFO's grill. Really, girl, that's not the best way to get a raise, at least not a financial one.

You might think this is one of the lesser offenses in this book, but I assure you it's not. It's actually a pretty major and common professional faux pas. In fact, when I do consulting work for major corporations, the human resources department will inevitably ask me to address it, especially with new hires. It seems fresh-out-of-college types have no idea that what's cute at spring break isn't so cool in the cubicle.

First of all, beware of low-rise pants at the office. Your trousers should really sit on the hip, not below it, while at work. And test out your top. If you're not tucking it in, your blouse should hang at least a few inches past your waistband while you're standing. This should give you enough room to reach down and pick things up without an ass-flash. Try it out at home, just to be safe.

And remember: A lady bends at the knee, even if she's very, very flexible.

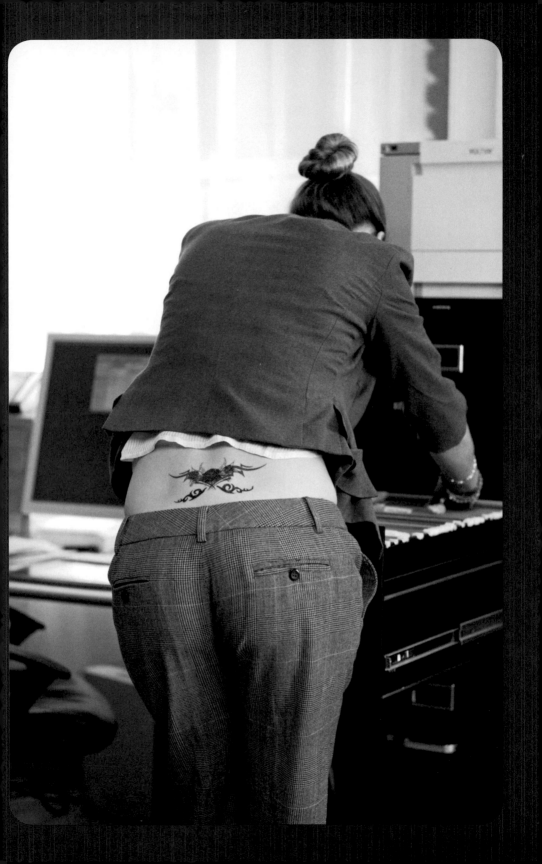

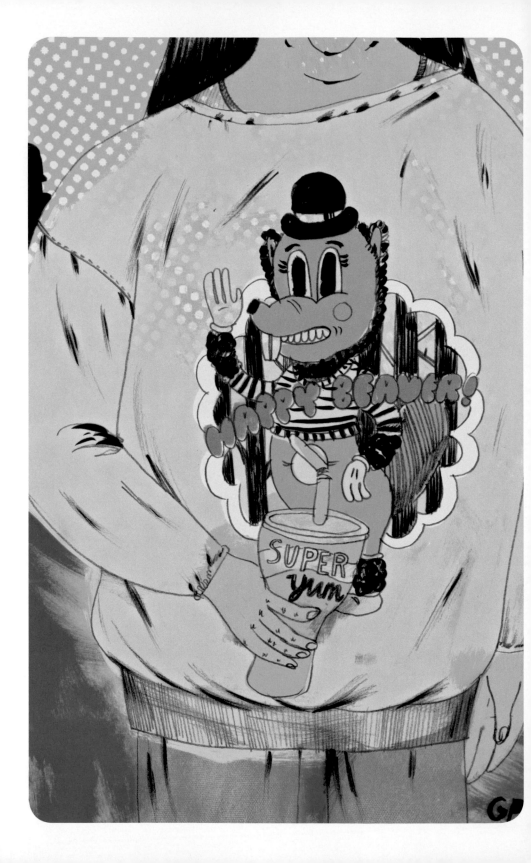

cartoon characters

Let's pretend you're at a party and you notice a handsome man standing in the kitchen. He's wearing a well-tailored suit and polished Italian shoes. His hair is clean and combed. His jaw is square and he has dimples like Jeff Probst. *Would you look at that,* you think. *That gorgeous guy is all alone. I feel bad for him. I'll be polite and strike up a conversation.* So you refresh your cocktail, discreetly check to make sure you have no lipstick on your teeth, and head over to him.

"What are you drinking?" you ask, hoping to break the ice gently.

"Grape juice," he says.

You laugh. "Oh, you mean red wine."

He stares at you blankly. "No. Grape juice. Want some?"

"Ummm . . . no thanks," you reply. "I'm okay." *Maybe he's an alkie.* You try to recover: "Seen any good movies lately?" A little clichéd, but you were thrown by the grape juice.

"I have *The Little Mermaid* on DVD. That's my favorite. I've seen it twenty-three times."

"Oh, well, that's a good movie, but I haven't—"

"I like candy!"

"Candy. Sure. Candy is nice."

"Boys have a penis. Girls have a vagina."

"So I've heard . . ."

"Whoopsie. I just made boom-boom in my pants."

Crazy, right? Well, so is wearing a sweatshirt with a god-damn talking duck on it! You know, in this book I've been trying to provide useful tips for fixing style mistakes, but the only advice I can think of giving here is: Burn any garment sporting a cartoon character, then make an appointment with a shrink. You've obviously got some unresolved issues from childhood and you are a menace to society.

denim on denim

Some people in the Pacific Northwest refer to it as the Canadian Tuxedo. In the rest of America they call it the Texas Tuxedo. In my house, I call it "the evil of which we do not speak"—denim on denim.

As I write this, a major retailer (the name of which rhymes with The Schmap) is trying to brainwash you into thinking that a denim shirt worn with denim jeans is stylish. I'm here to tell you that if you look like the models in the advertising campaign, you could wear a halfway decomposed dead antelope on your back and people would still line up around the block to have sex with you. But denim on denim is not a good look on 99.99 percent of the population. (Let's face it, though; it's hot as hell on a good-looking cowboy.)

Quite frankly, there is no woman less stylish than the chick at the mall wearing a denim shirt and light-wash jeans with crappy white sneakers, a bad perm, and a scrunchie. If this describes you, I need you to know that you are my nemesis and I will do everything in my power to destroy you.

You may wear jeans, of course. You may wear a denim jacket.

Just don't wear them together !!!

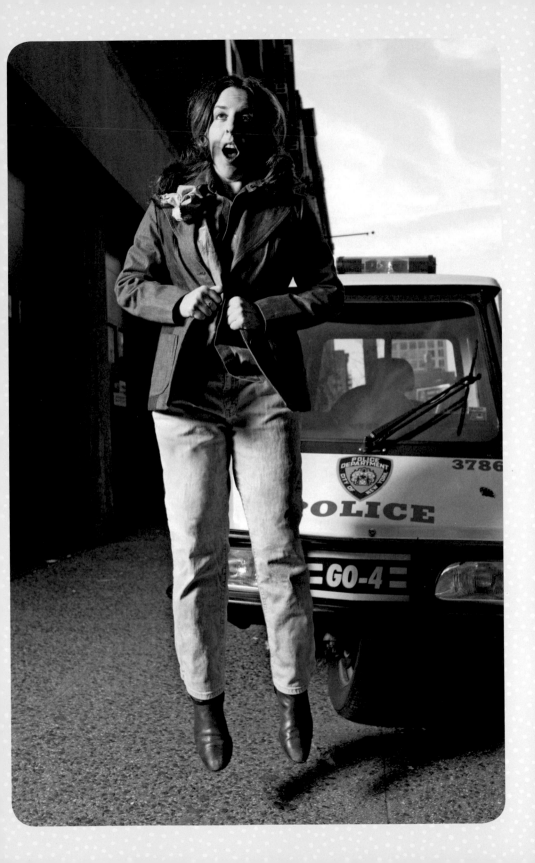

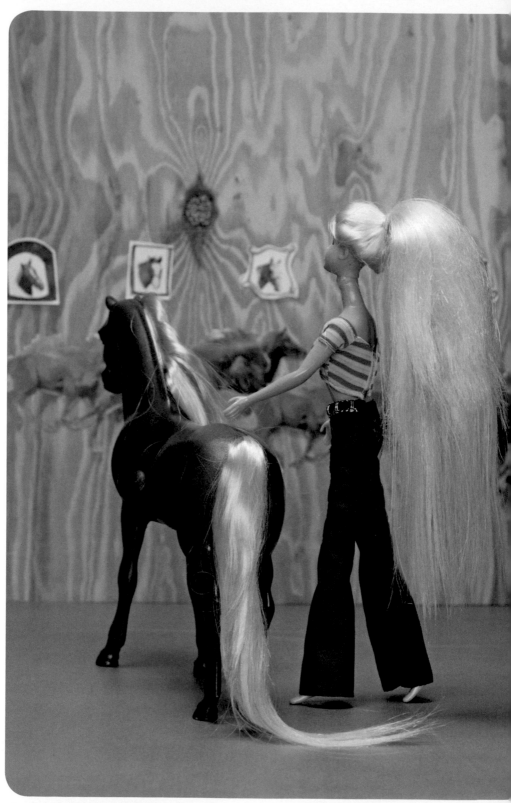

horse hair

"My husband likes my hair long, so I haven't cut it since we got married in 1974. I do everything my husband tells me to do anyway. You know, things like shining his big belt buckles and making sure there's always at least three cartons of unfiltered cigarettes in the cab of his truck. It's how we express our love for each other. I do little things for him and he doesn't hit me in front of my parents. And I don't care that Crystal Gayle hasn't had a number one song since 'Don't It Make My Brown Eyes Blue'; she's still my style icon. So, so pretty. Conditioner? Never heard of it. Is that like shining the leaves of my philodendron with a little mayonnaise on a damp paper towel? Because I do that sometimes."

My dear reader, when it comes to improving your style, who are you going to trust, me or your husband? He might be a nice guy, but he's hardly impartial. He's got a boatload of issues that involve you, either directly or indirectly. I, on the other hand, have only your best interest in mind, always. Clinton loves you unconditionally. Especially if you paid full price for this book.

And so, I'm here to tell you that after a certain age—let's say, thirty—ultralong, styleless hair makes you appear to be desperately hanging onto your youth or your man or both. Yes, *desperate*. And desperation is never cute.

Don't get me wrong: I'm not saying you need a chin-length bob or Grandma's hair helmet, but you do need a hairstyle. Maybe a few layers here and there just to keep things interesting and modern, not to mention more flattering. Regular upkeep of your hair is just as important to your appearance as maintaining healthy teeth and gums, keeping your nose free of boogers, and plucking those bristles off your chin. Go make a hair appointment. Now. And please don't tell your husband I was talking smack about him. He scares me.

socks with clogs

I think it's pretty safe to say that the kind of woman who wears socks with clogs is not reading this book. That's because the woman who wears socks with clogs hasn't heard of me. Instead of watching reality television, she spends her time herding goats, making candles, and bickering with her husband's other wives.

The only exceptions to the no-socks-with-clogs rule are for registered nurses in the ER, when paired with scrubs; gardeners in the privacy of their own backyards; and Mario Batali when he's behind the stove. Other than that, just don't do it. Now go back to the commune and spread the word.

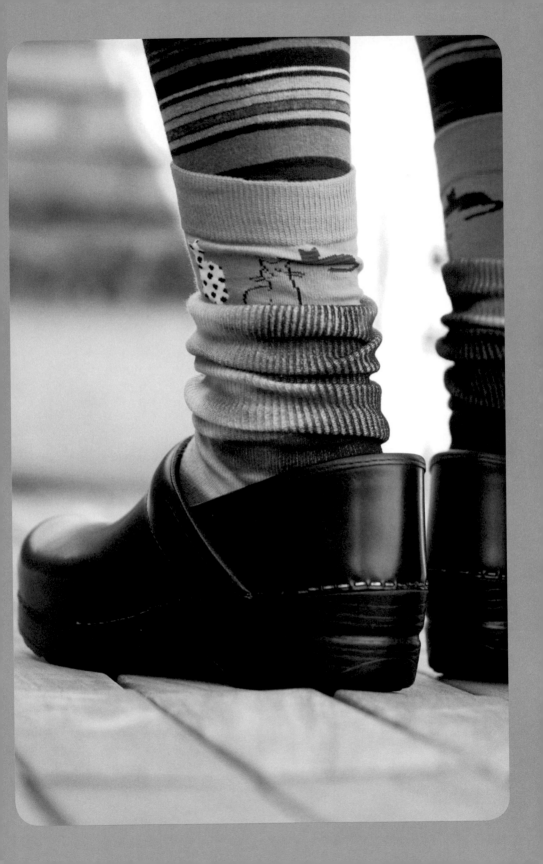

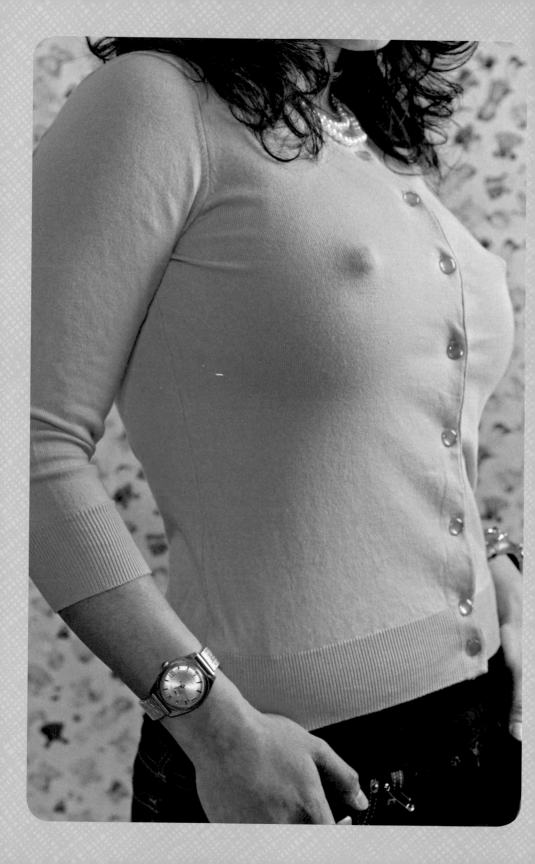

nipping out

Nothing pulls focus like a set of high beams. Whether you're delivering a speech on quantum physics to a bunch of MIT nerds or discussing your favorite brownie recipe with the other members of the baking club, when your nippies scream yippee, you've lost your audience. All attention's on the ta-tas.

This is nothing to be ashamed of. It's just how the human body works. But following the same logic, you can't expect people not to look. We're drawn to boobs!

So, if you're the type who springs to attention any time someone cranks up the AC or when Gerard Butler walks into the room, be prepared, especially when wearing a thin knit top. A padded bra will diminish the impact for most women, or you can insert silicone petals between you and your cups.

Just hurry. Before someone loses an eye.

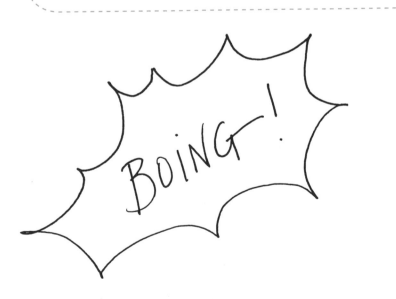

black addiction

If more than 50 percent of your wardrobe is black, you are most likely deluding yourself into thinking that:

- **BLACK IS SLIMMING.** Not necessarily. A white jacket that fits you well is more slimming than a black shapeless hoodie.

- **BLACK IS FLATTERING.** Not on older or imperfect skin. Black increases the appearance of under-eye circles, wrinkles, blackheads, and facial scars.

- **BLACK IS TOUGH, COOL, AND/OR SOPHISTICATED.** Sure, I'll give you that one. It's hard to look like a complete bitch in mint green, though sometimes Nancy Pelosi pulls it off.

I often find that women who wear only black don't feel too great about their bodies and use black as urban camouflage. I hate to break it to you, but black doesn't make you invisible. Clothes that fit you well can trick others into thinking you have a better body than you actually do and, perhaps more important, lend an air of self-respect to your appearance. Focus on fit before color.

Also, after a certain age, consider replacing black with softer neutrals, like navy, brown, or gray, which are exponentially easier on the complexion. Is black okay for evening attire at any age? Of course, because women usually wear more makeup at night to cover up imperfections, and the lights are also dimmer.

Black is absolutely classic and often sophisticated, but best when used in moderation. Let it help you be chic, but don't let it become your schtick.

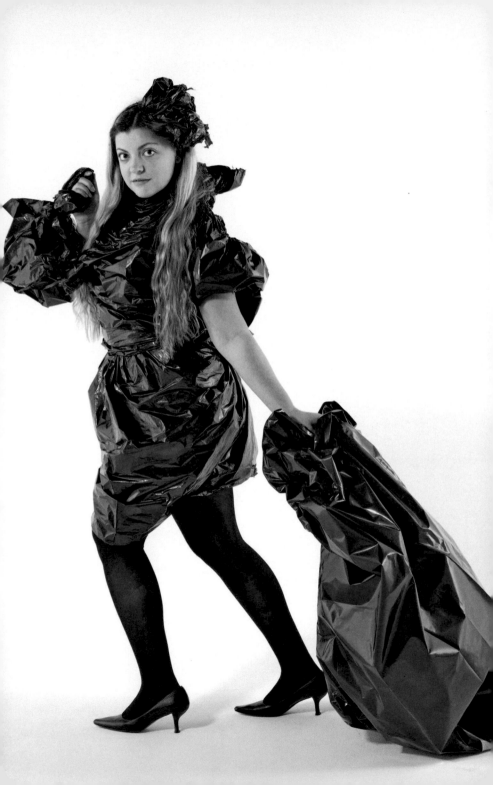

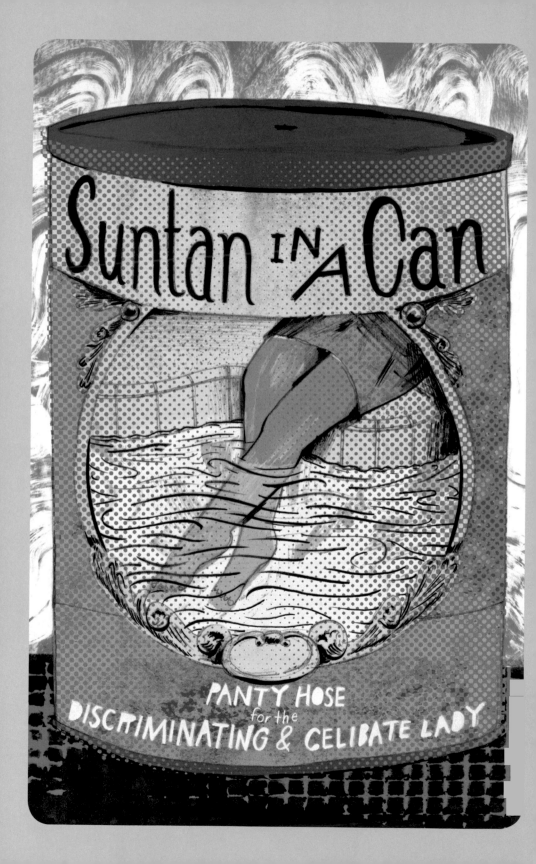

suntan hose

I hate to break it to you, but suntan hose will not make you look like you have a suntan. They will make you look like you lost circulation in your lower extremities while Reagan was still in office.

The key to wearing hosiery successfully is to look like you're *not* wearing any hosiery—or to look like you *are* wearing hosiery. (If that's not the most profound thing you've heard all day, you are too smart to be reading this book.) In other words, buy a shade that matches your natural skin tone as closely as possible. Or . . . wear an opaque, colored, patterned, or textured pair of hose.

My next book will be about how to perform brain surgery on oneself.

turtlenecks

Your neck is important for several reasons: It houses the conduits that bring blood to your brain and nerve signals to your body. It plays a pretty big role in swallowing and breathing. And it deserves to be seen.

If you've got a naturally thin or long neck, you can disregard this section. But if you have a short or thick neck, a turtleneck is one of the least flattering things you can wear. Visually elongating the neck is one of the simplest tricks for visually elongating yourself. That is, make the neck appear longer and you appear longer. When you appear longer, you appear leaner. So, conversely, when you shorten your neck by adding bulk to it, you end up looking shorter and squatter.

You're much better off wearing V-necks, which open up and elongate the neck. And don't give me any crap about your neck getting cold. The solution is called a scarf. Look into it.

Frumpy, dumpy, and lumpy makes me GRUMPY.

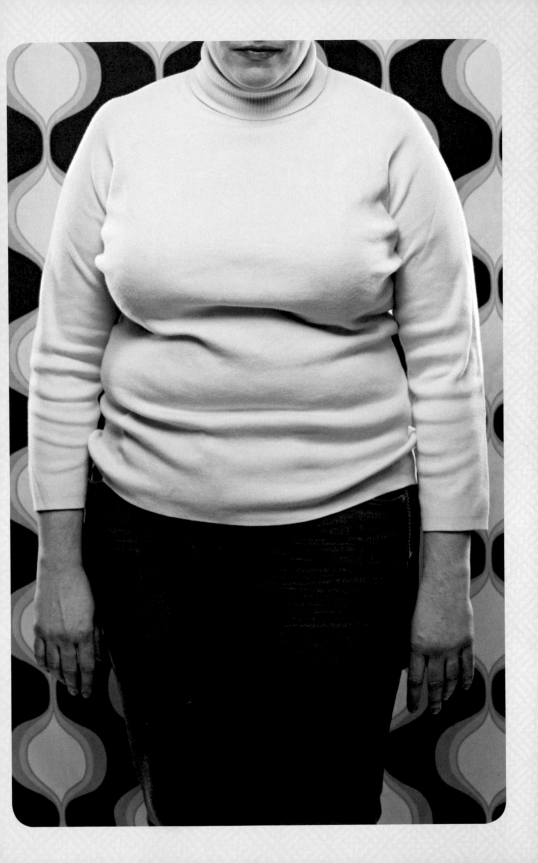

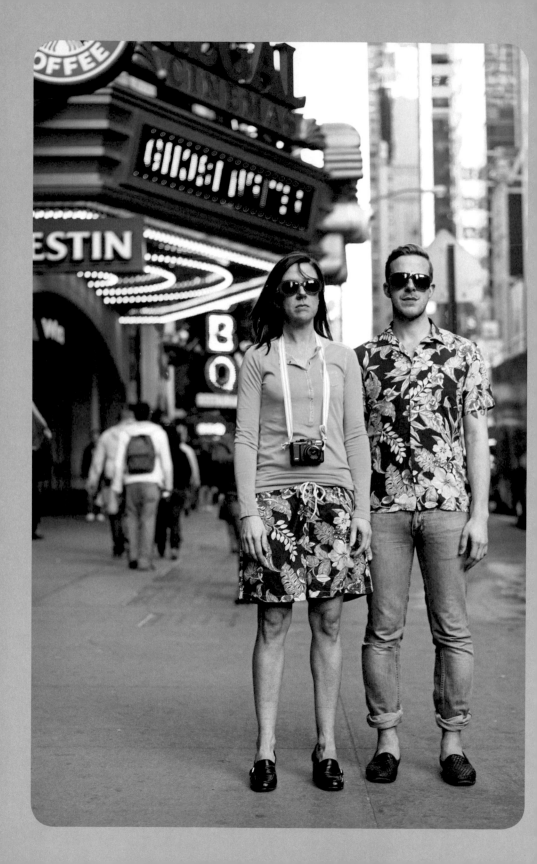

matching your mate

Any heterosexual American man willing to wear clothing identical to yours is probably a serial killer—unless you convinced him to do so by withholding sex; then he's just whipped.

I don't care if you think it's cute to wear matching aloha shirts on a cruise or if you found the same reindeer sweater for your Christmas card. I'm here to tell you that the rest of us are posting pictures of you on our blogs and adding captions like "When cousins marry."

I'm not saying you can't coordinate, because you can. That means dressing to the same level, like instead of a guy wearing jeans and a T-shirt to a dinner party when his wife is wearing a cocktail dress, he wears trousers and a blazer. And if her dress is pink, he can wear a shirt that has a faint pink stripe. Nothing too obvious; it doesn't have to be the exact same shade of pink or a solid pink shirt, just a touch. Sometimes that's nice. Don't force it, though!

I'm going to cut same-sex couples a little slack on this one. If you're the same size as your wife or girlfriend, of course you should heed the call to double your wardrobe. But know that sharing clothes increases your chances of looking like lesbian twins. Believe it or not, I don't know a lot of lesbians, probably because I don't live in Brooklyn, so I had to ask my friend Kera, who does live in Brooklyn, what's up. She said, "Sometimes you just aspire to be like your girlfriend, but one of you does it better. It's an occupational hazard of nesting and cohabitation, and of laundry and desperation."

Oh, that's cute. I'm going to make a point to befriend more lezzies.

the monica shoe

I was never a big fan of *Friends*. I don't know why. Actually, I do know why. David Schwimmer. Nevertheless, one night a few years ago, I was in some hotel room, somewhere, unable to sleep. So I turned on the telly. I could have watched an infomercial about colon cleansing for the seventy-fifth time, but nooooo, I had to watch a rerun of *Friends*. I couldn't even tell you what the episode was about, but the plot went something like this: Ross loves Rachel! Rachel is confused! Monica, you're such a neat freak! Joey is stupid! So is Phoebe! The other guy is a smart-ass! Let's be friends forever!

It's a good thing I forgot to bring my sleeping pills on that trip because I would have chugged them like a box of Nerds. Anyway, during all the scintillating hubbub, I saw it! Right there on Courteney Cox's feet! The clunky, chunky, black, square-toe shoe, the origin of which I had been trying to pinpoint for years! I mean, I used to wonder, *Why? Why, God, do so many women own these shoes?!* But right then, I realized, it's Monica. That skinny raven-haired sous chef started it!

Let me tell you, ladies, if you want to gain five pounds instantly, wear that shoe. A clunky, chunky shoe will always make you look clunky and chunky. Granted, it didn't make Courteney look chunky because she weighs eighty-seven pounds right out of the shower. But I do think it's the reason she always looked a little exasperated. She was dragging those heavy feet around all day.

When I style a woman, my goal is that when I'm done she'll look like she's hovering a hairbreadth above the ground as she walks across the room. That's hard to do with cement blocks on your feet, so buy shoes that have a visual lightness to them. Maybe a paler color, or something metallic. Perhaps strappy or woven, like an espadrille. If it's light in your hand, you'll look lighter in it.

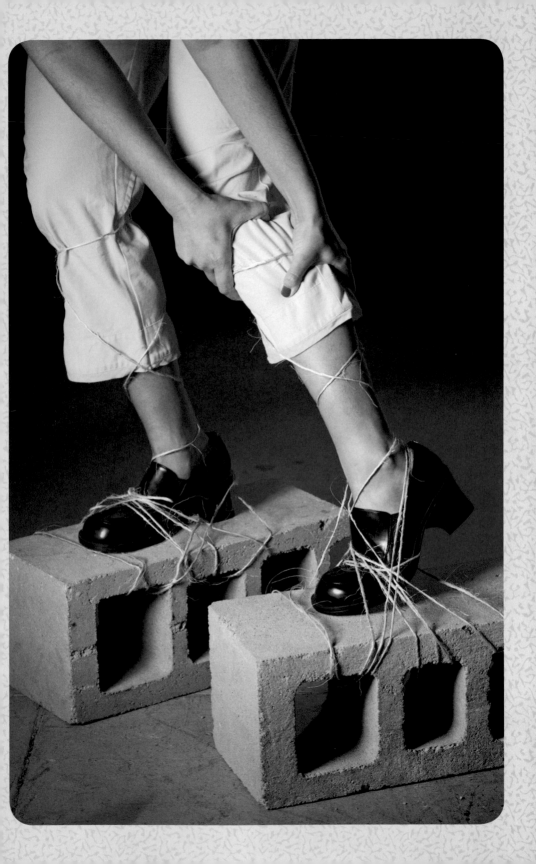

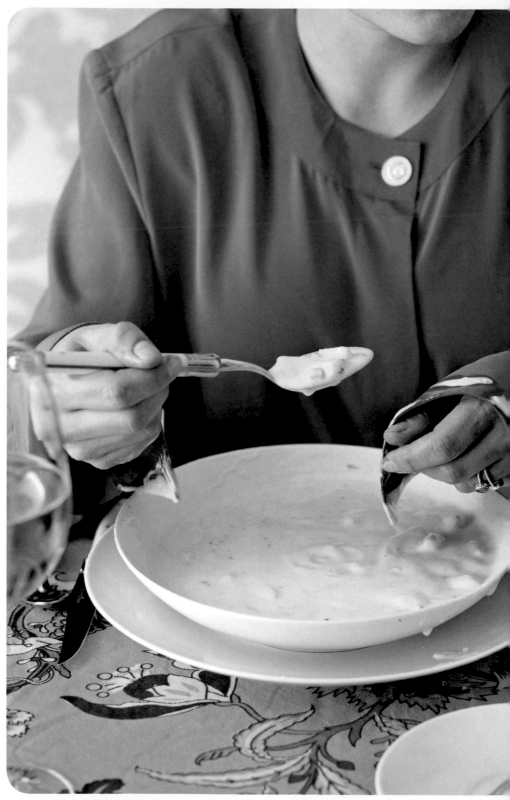

too-long sleeves

Is the too-long sleeve the worst style faux pas in the world? Nope. But my favorite thing about you is your distaste for mediocrity. You don't buy piecrust, you make it from scratch. When you vacuum the house, you move the furniture. When you paint a wall, you prime it first. When a cop gives you a speeding ticket, you say, "Thank you, Officer. Have a nice day." So why would you settle for sleeves that cover your hands? You wouldn't!

Look at your hand. See that muscle under your thumb? (It's called your opponens pollicis.) When your arms are held by your sides, your long-sleeve blouse should hit the middle of that muscle. (FYI: A man's long sleeve is generally a little shorter, hitting where the wrist meets the hand.) When a sleeve covers more of your hand, you start to look like a little kid who borrowed her mom's shirt for art class.

It's a pretty simple alteration. A tailor can remove some of the sleeve but keep all of the cuff. Or you can take the easy way out and roll up your sleeves. But we'd both know you'd be cheating.

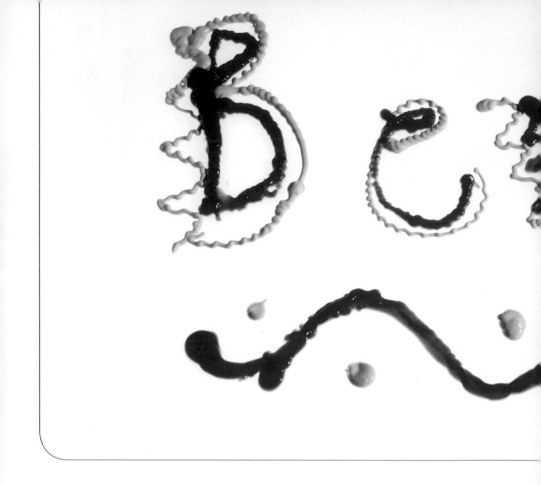

condiment colors

People ask me all the time: "What colors should I wear?"

I think they expect me to say something like, "Well, because you're an Arctic Winter with undertones of Parisian Spring, you should stick to a palette of mauve and chartreuse."

It doesn't work like that, people! The whole seasonal color thing is a load of hooey. Somebody made about three billion bucks off the concept and good for them. To be honest, I wish I had thought of it, because I'd be writing this book from Tahiti instead of on a flight to Houston.

Wear the colors that make you happy. But beware of the condiments!

Ketchup red is often a bad color for people with pink skin—whether that's an overall pink tone because you're of Nordic, Anglo, or Ger-

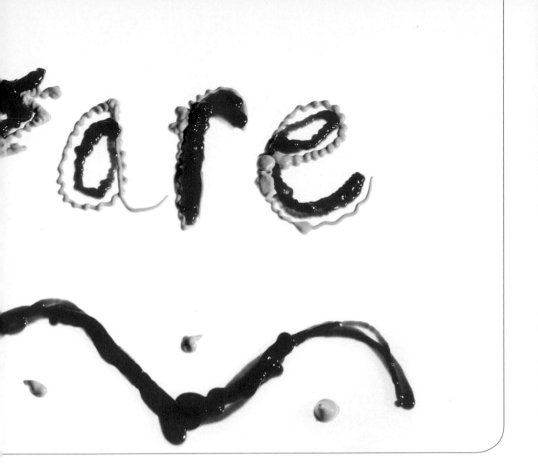

manic descent, or because you have pinkish-red splotchy skin due to eczema, acne, or broken capillaries. Wearing red near your face will only visually exacerbate these imperfections.

Mustard yellow is a tricky color for people whose skin has yellow undertones—often people of Asian, African, Hispanic, or Middle Eastern descent. Mustard yellow will bring out the yellow already present in your face, making you look like you have a liver condition.

When reds have blue undertones, they are easier to wear. Some yellows are bright and don't make skin look jaundiced. And, of course, expertly applied makeup is probably the best way to fix imperfect skin, which would allow you to wear just whatever colors you want.

So wear what makes you feel pretty. Who's in the mood for a hot dog?

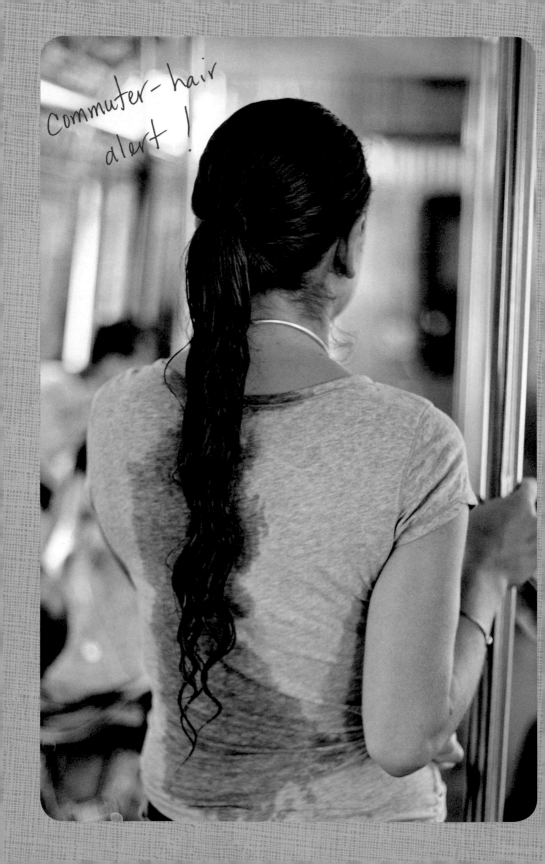

wet hair ponytail

Are you really showing up to work like that? With your hair all slicked back around your head and some half-assed assemblage of wet noodles dangling behind you? I'm sorry, does your house not have electricity? Did you miss the invention of that little gizmo called the blow-dryer? And why are you fifteen minutes late for work every day? I think you have some time-management issues. Here's an idea: Set the alarm for twenty minutes earlier in the morning and stop staying up so late at night in chat rooms discussing why you think Mario Lopez should be your boyfriend.

the whale tail

About ten years ago, when I was working as a magazine editor, there was a period when all the office interns would come into work with their thong straps sticking out of the top of their jeans. I thought it was stupid then, and I think it's moronic now. These days, the only women who think this look is sexy are thirteen-year-olds and hillbillies. And thirteen-year-old hillbillies.

Pull your jeans up and tuck your straps in. We get it; you're wearing a thong. Now, stop kissing your brother and go see the dentist.

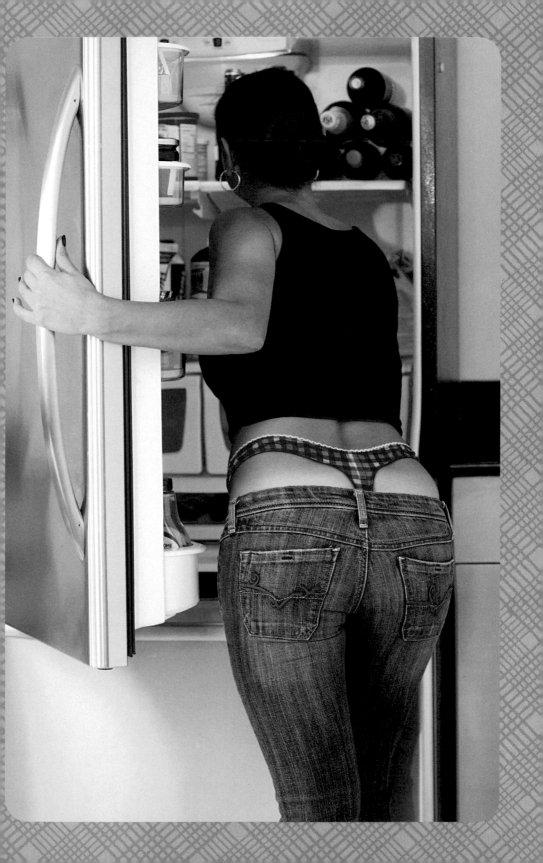

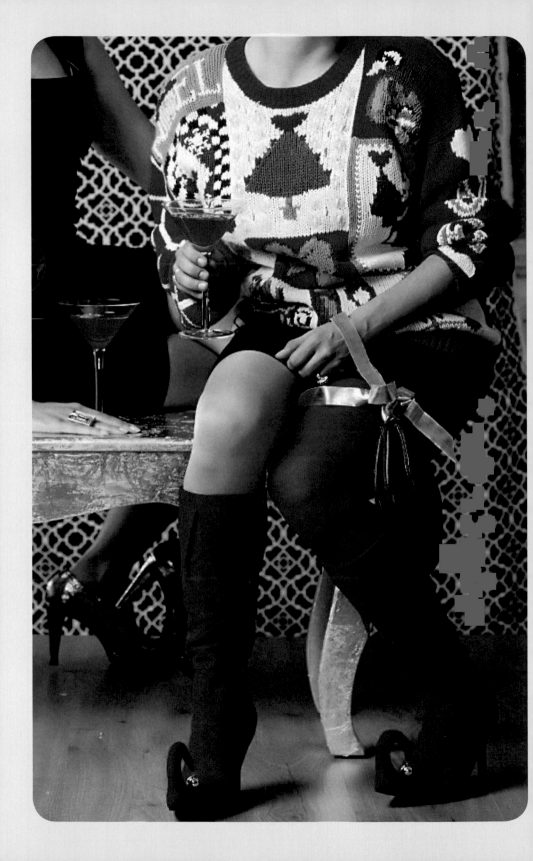

holiday sweaters

You're wearing a holiday sweater! Wow. Use this flow chart to find out what it says about you!

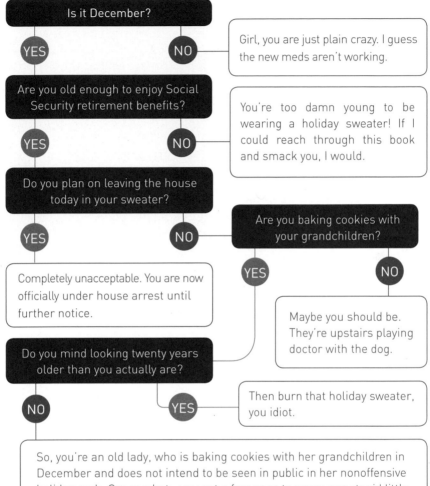

Is it December?

YES / **NO** → Girl, you are just plain crazy. I guess the new meds aren't working.

Are you old enough to enjoy Social Security retirement benefits?

YES / **NO** → You're too damn young to be wearing a holiday sweater! If I could reach through this book and smack you, I would.

Do you plan on leaving the house today in your sweater?

YES → Completely unacceptable. You are now officially under house arrest until further notice.

NO → **Are you baking cookies with your grandchildren?**

YES / **NO** → Maybe you should be. They're upstairs playing doctor with the dog.

Do you mind looking twenty years older than you actually are?

YES → Then burn that holiday sweater, you idiot.

NO → So, you're an old lady, who is baking cookies with her grandchildren in December and does not intend to be seen in public in her nonoffensive holiday garb. Guess what—you get a free pass to wear your stupid little sweater. Pat yourself on the back; you beat the system. Happy holidays. Excuse me while I pee on that snowman in your front yard.

Now, for the rest of you: If you want to dress stylishly for the holidays, try a cashmere sweater, perhaps one with an embellished neckline. Or how about a cluster of antique brooches on the lapel of a velvet jacket. Or better yet, if you want to spread holiday cheer, just say things like "Merry Christmas!" or "Happy Hanukkah!" or "Joyous Kwanzaa!" Or just give people money. That's the true spirit of the season.

too much cleavage at work

I think it's important to maintain an air of professionalism in the office at all times . . . which is why I haven't worked in an office for almost a decade. On a television set, you can curse and talk about sex and drugs and let the bodily functions fly, and no one gets pissed off. In fact, they give you your own series for shit like that.

But if you work in some kind of corporate environment, it's probably best to play by the rules. And rule number one is: Keep the boobies under control. The general rule of thumb is: YES TO CHEST, NO TO BREAST. In other words, make sure the soft tissue is covered.

Buy a few camisoles and wear 'em. While you're at it, keep your shoulders covered at work and hemlines to the knee. *Ally McBeal* got canceled for a reason. And it wasn't just the ridiculous plotlines and overexposure of that dancing baby.

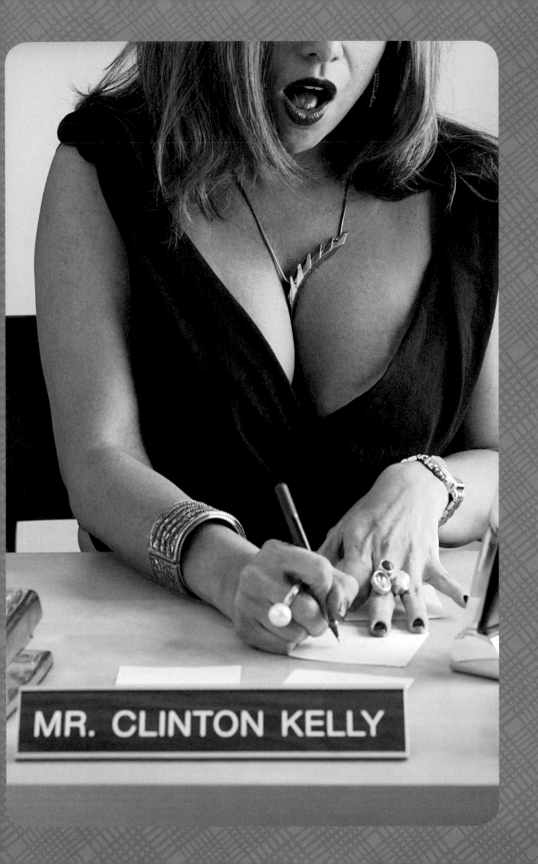

MR. CLINTON KELLY

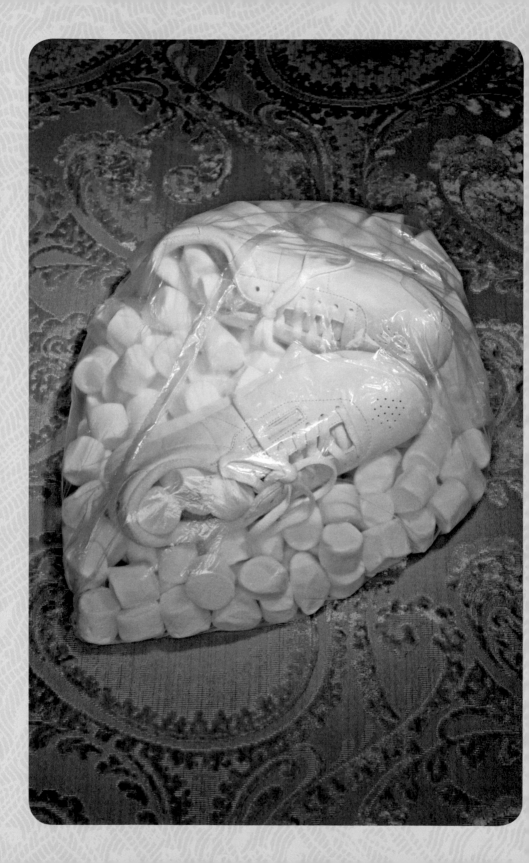

cross-trainers

Richard Simmons called. He wants his sneakers back. No, he really did call. He was also wondering when he could pick up his Right Said Fred CD.

I'm not gonna lie . . . well, at least not about this: Cross-trainers, when worn as casual footwear, are the bane of my existence. I mean, they really, really, *really* piss me off. I guess you could say they make me cross.

Why? Oh, I suppose it's because they epitomize "middle-of-the-road" and a complete disregard for style in general. And they always seem to be worn by people who exercise rarely. At most.

If you are actively participating in a step class or watching a Tae Bo video or working as a gymnastics coach, I might be able to tolerate this comfort shoe. But you're not. You're at the mall! You're at the airport! You're at the dentist! You are everywhere *except* at the gym!

Let's get a few things straight: I don't mind sneakers. The world is full of really fabulous ones. Athletic sneakers help you better perform your sport of choice. Maybe they have little air pumps or springs or ankle support. Thrilling. Wear them while exercising. When you're done exercising, take them off and put on a freakin' shoe.

If you want a comfortable shoe, you can look for a non-athletic sneaker. This is a sneaker designed to be cute and comfortable but is not suited for, say, running a marathon. They come in pretty colors and fun styles. Oh, joy.

Other comfortable shoe options include:

- **FLATS.** Now, there's an idea!
- **BOOTS.** Groundbreaking.
- **SANDALS.** Can you believe how smart I am?

Okay, Clinton, deep breath. In through the nose, out through the mouth. Life is too short for me to care about this. YET I DO! Where are my pills?

frayed hems

When I see a woman walking down the sidewalk with pants so long they're all ripped up and dragging on the ground, I think: *She's lazy. It would have taken a tailor twenty minutes and ten bucks to hem those things.* Then I begin to wonder what kind of filthy city residue those too-long pants are Swiffering along the way. Maybe a little dried-up dog poo and some homeless guy's phlegm. Then I wonder what kind of person doesn't care about carrying all those germs into her house! She's probably the type who sleeps on a mattress without a fitted sheet and who has a lot of wax in her ears! Then I throw up a little in my mouth, because earwax makes me sick.

A lot of people think you can't hem jeans, but a lot of people are wrong. Ask your tailor to maintain the original hem by cutting it off and reattaching it. This has become pretty standard practice, so if he looks at you like you're nuts, grab your jeans and run.

Sometimes the original hem can't be reattached, usually if the jeans have a bootcut or flared leg (because the leg opening is wider on the original hem than it will be once it is shortened). If this is the case, ask the tailor to add a stitch of gold thread about half an inch above the new hem. It'll look less like your mom hemmed your jeans for you and more like you bought them that way. You could even—if you're feeling crafty—lightly abrade the new hem with a little sandpaper to make it look less perfect.

How long should your jeans be? About a quarter of an inch off the ground, depending on what kind of shoe you're wearing. Sorry, but the same jeans usually won't work for both flats and heels. You're better off having separate pairs for different heel heights.

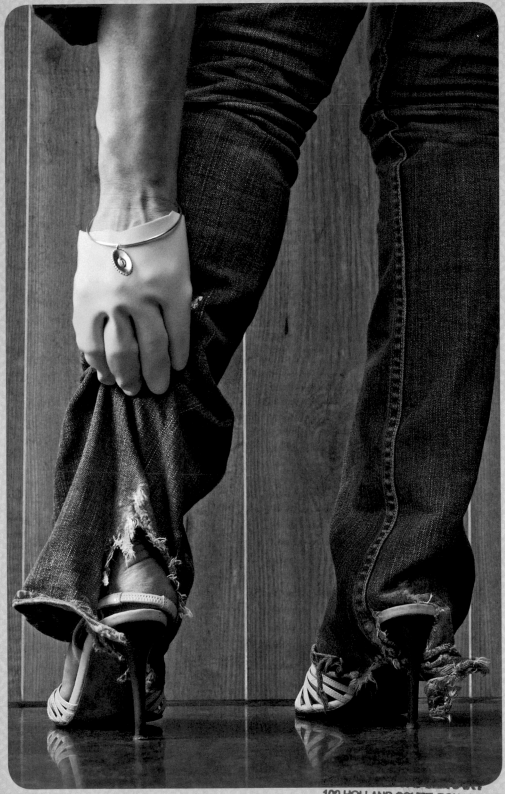

100 HOLLAND COURT, BOX 130
BRADFORD, ONT. L3Z 2A7

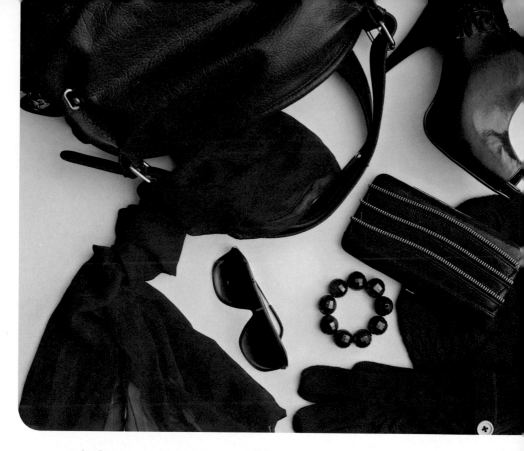

matchy-matchy outfits

I've heard so many people reminisce about Garanimals with longing and nostalgia. "Oh, life was so easy back then. You'd match the pants with the tiger tag to the top with the tiger tag and you'd be ready for school in no time! Man, those were the days."

Is it just me or is matching rust-orange corduroys to a rust-orange polo shirt about as difficult as picking your eight-year-old nose? I mean, come on. If you can't do this without the help of animal tags by the second grade, you need more than after-school tutoring.

Matching your top to your bottom makes you look simpleminded, completely out-of-date, or just plain old. Style has changed since the 1950s. It's not about wearing the perfectly matching set as it is displayed on a mannequin. It's about putting pieces together with your own twist.

Look, if you absolutely *love* a print that comes in both a blouse and a skirt, I suppose you could buy both pieces. But for the love of Lagerfeld, **DO NOT WEAR THEM TOGETHER.**

I know many women have a difficult time matching pieces, and that's because things don't need to "match," they need to "go." For example, forest green and sage green don't match, but they go, so you can wear a sage green sweater with a forest green suede boot. Another example is gold and yellow; they don't match, but you could wear a blouse that has some gold in the print with jeans and a yellow flat.

Speaking of jeans, they're neutral, so any color or print works with denim. Other neutrals are black, gray, navy, brown, khaki, and white. Technically, any color goes with any neutral, and all neutrals go with each other. Some colors and neutrals pair better than others. A few combinations don't work so well:

BLACK + ORANGE = *Halloween*

GREEN + ORANGE = *Pumpkin*

BLACK + YELLOW = *Bumblebee*

RED + GREEN = *Christmas*

And you may be wondering whether you can wear black and navy together or black and brown. The answer is yes and yes. The key to making both of those neutral combinations work is *intention.* A very dark navy blue that looks almost black paired with actual black will make it seem like you got dressed in the dark. But a lighter navy can be paired with black without a problem.

Black and brown have a similar relationship. Very dark chocolate brown is harder to pair with black than, say, a milk-chocolate brown. And I've found that the best way to combine black and brown is by using a print that contains both neutrals. Maybe you've got an abstract geometric-print blouse that contains purple, black, and brown. You could wear it with black trousers (because there's black in the print) and a brown jacket (because there's also brown in the print).

When a woman tells me that she is absolutely hopeless at putting outfits together and still cannot grasp the concept of "going," I advise her to keep all her bottoms neutral. If she owns:

- A BLACK PENCIL SKIRT
- GRAY TROUSERS
- DARK-WASH JEANS
- KHAKIS
- AND/OR WHITE WALKING SHORTS

she'll be hard-pressed to find a top that doesn't go with at least one of those bottoms.

red lipstick

Some women's magazines will tell you that red lipstick is the sexiest thing a woman can wear. When I was a women's magazine editor, I think I may have even written a headline like: "Seduce your man when he comes home from work! Surprise him by wearing red lips and nothing else!" What can I say? It was a job and I needed the money. It was either that or sell crack.

I'd like to officially apologize and inform you that red lipstick is just a plain old bad choice for some gals. Look, if your mouth is not your best feature, a thick coat of cherry red lipstick will not magically make it so. This might sound harsh, but Uncle Clinty is just telling you the truth. Think twice about red lipstick if:

- your mouth is disproportionately large for your face
- your teeth are crooked
- your teeth are yellow, brown, or missing
- your lips are really thin

If any of the above apply, don't get down on yourself. That's not the point. You should be accentuating your *best* feature, not bringing all the attention to your second best or your worst. If your mouth isn't perfect, why let it steal the show? Play up your eyes, your cheekbones, your skin quality, your hair, whatever.

But if you insist upon bright reds, my friend Carmindy, makeup artist extraordinaire, says that blue-based lip colors will make your teeth look whiter. That doesn't mean wear blue lipstick. "Blue-based means cooler in tone. Think of it as the difference between fuchsia, which is blue-based, and fire-engine red."

I say red lipstick is overrated and should be used occasionally at best. When I'm talking to a woman wearing bright red lipstick, all I can look at is her mouth, which soon starts to take on a life of its own. Then I think of the opening sequence of *The Rocky Horror Picture Show* and I haven't got the slightest idea what she's saying. I can only picture her wearing garters and dancing the Time Warp.

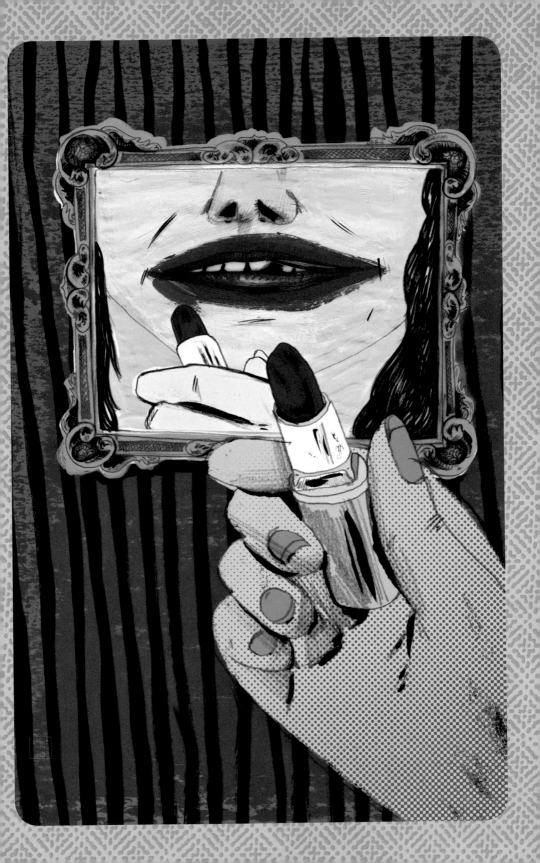

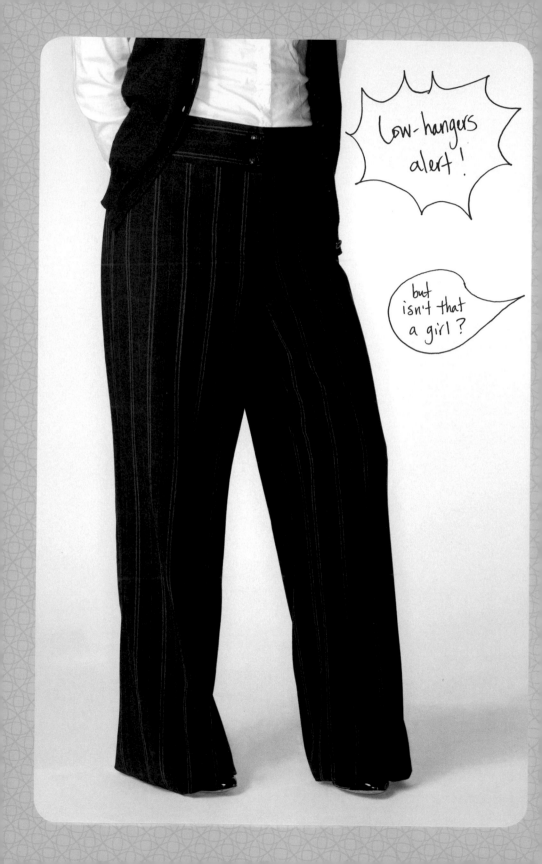

dropped crotch

When you're out in public, you don't want the first thing people notice about you to be your woowoo. You might want them to think: *What pretty eyes she has.* Or, *Mmmm, she smells nice.* Or, *I wonder where she got those shoes.* But most respectable women I know don't want complete strangers wondering, *Why is that lady's crotch hanging down to her knees?*

Ideally, the crotch of your pants should rest pretty darn close to your own anatomical crotch. When it doesn't, it either becomes a distraction (see Camel Toe, page 114, and The Little Nubbin in the Boat, page 172) or it shortens the line of the leg. I'll explain: One of the visual cues we use to judge the leg length of others is the distance between the crotch and the hem of the pant. If the crotch is a couple of inches lower than it should be, your legs look two inches shorter. When your legs look shorter, you look shorter. When you look shorter, you look wider.

And so the reverse is true. (Wow, this is starting to sound a lot like math.) Raise the crotch and the legs look longer. If the legs look longer, you look taller. When you look taller, you look thinner.

Generally, the crotch of a pant will hang too low for one of two reasons: 1. The pants are too loose in the waist and are sliding down the hip, or 2. The woman is a petite from the waist down but is wearing pants cut for a taller woman. And so the fixes are these: 1. Have the pants taken in at the waist, and they will sit where they should on the hip and crotch. 2. If you are petite, your first stop when shopping—especially for pants—should be the petites department. Petite is generally defined as five foot four or shorter. However, in my experience, some women who are up to five foot six might need to shop in petites for pants if they are long-waisted (or for tops if they are short-waisted). This doesn't mean that you will always have to shop in the petites department if you are petite, but your chances of finding a proper fit off the rack will be greater. If you're a petite and you do want to shop in the missy (regular) department, look for pants marked low-rise or mid-rise first and expect your pants to need hemming.

Note: Harem pants (loose-fitting pants with an intentionally dropped crotch) became trendy for about three minutes while I was writing this book. I don't find them particularly flattering on anyone, but you should feel free to wear them if you enjoy looking like a grown woman walking around with a full diaper. Or if it's Hammertime!

beige

I hate beige. Nobody looks good in beige. Well, almost nobody.

Beige and its first cousins, tan and khaki, are valuable neutrals, without a doubt. Khaki pants are a great casual option for just about everyone, as long as they fit and flatter your body. And a cute little tan cotton canvas jacket? Adorable. But worn without color by the face, these light neutrals can make your skin look drab, sallow, lifeless, or ruddy. Here's why:

Anytime you wear a color near your face, you are automatically establishing a relationship between your face and the color. For example, let's say you're like me and have the average white person's complexion. If I were to wear, say, a beige turtleneck, you would look at me and, without even realizing you're doing it, compare the color of my shirt to the color of my face. The turtleneck, being a manufactured garment, would be pretty uniform in its quality, color, and texture. My face, however, is not. So you would be much more likely to notice a few sunspots on my forehead, some broken capillaries near my nose, maybe a little razor burn on my chin, and some wrinkles near my eyes. (Yikes!)

If you have darker skin, beige isn't going to present the same problem. In fact, if you've got very dark skin, beige might offer a great contrast. But for the most part, people with light to medium tones won't be flattered by beige unless it's paired with a little bright color by the face.

However, if you have perfect skin and it's one of your best qualities, go right ahead and wear colors that are close to your skin tone. People will look at your top and make a favorable comparison: "Oh, look, her skin is just as perfect as that off-white cashmere crewneck. How does she do it?" (For more tips on color, see Condiment Colors, page 56.)

Now excuse me while I call to make an appointment for a facial.

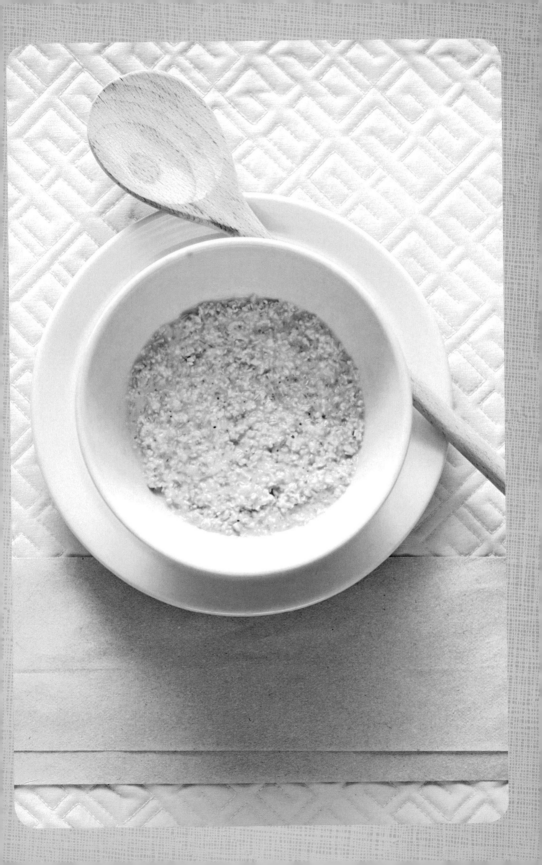

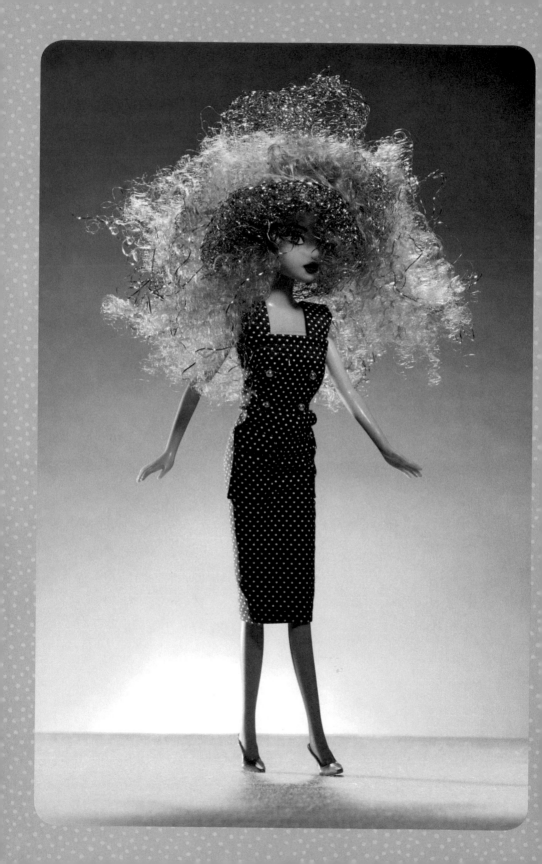

frizz

Some women can rock an ultrafrizzy head of hair. A few years ago, I had lunch at Harry Cipriani, and Diana Ross was at the next table. Her hair was literally wider than her chair. It was a-maaaaa-zing, and I wanted to get lost in it. Literally. I fantasized that if I crawled inside I would be transported into a parallel universe. I used to wish the same thing when I watched *Mister Rogers' Neighborhood,* that I would crawl into that hole in the wall and follow the trolley into the Neighborhood of Make-Believe. I guess that's what Diana Ross's hair was like for me, a portal to a magical land where people wear designer clothes and birds poop sedatives. For example, you might find a little yellow pill on the hood of your car right after you wash it, or you could be outside on a sunny day and feel something drop right on the top of your head. And when you touch your hair you realize it's two Xanax.

That's the land I want to live in, and it's in Diana Ross's hair. So, my point is . . . hold on, it'll come to me . . . Oh yeah, if you have frizz-prone hair, you must either:

1. Go with the frizz and *own* it, like La Ross

or

2. Smooth it out

or

3. Turn the frizz into curls

A huge head of frizzy hair can be a superchic accessory, but it requires confidence to wear around town—and it's got to be the right shape. So find a hairstylist who specializes in big, curly hair and knows how to cut it.

If you're not going with the fro, you've got to tame the beast. Half-assed frizz makes it look like your hair's running the show, not you. So look for products that will coerce your coif into distinct curls. (This may involve the use of a diffuser.) Or start honing your flat-iron skills for a sleeker look.

Whatever you choose, commit to it! And if you're ever at Harry Cipriani, get the risotto. Yum!

horizontal stripes

As a stylist, I am constantly striving to create the illusion of height. Not because I think you should look taller. Quite frankly, I don't care how tall you are. But most women I've worked with want to look thinner, and when you appear taller you appear thinner. Think of a woman who weighs 150 pounds. That woman would appear very different at five foot two than she would at five foot ten. So it stands to reason that if you can visually stretch yourself vertically, like a comic strip character imprinted on Silly Putty, you'll lose visual poundage.

When you wear horizontal stripes, you are fighting against verticality, making yourself appear wider. That said, however, some women can wear horizontal stripes without issue because they are tall or thin or both. This is why looks on the runway don't necessarily translate to real women. When a model is six feet tall and weighs 100 pounds, she doesn't need a visual stretch; she needs a sandwich.

If you want to look thinner, make people's eyes go this way ↑, not this way ←——→.

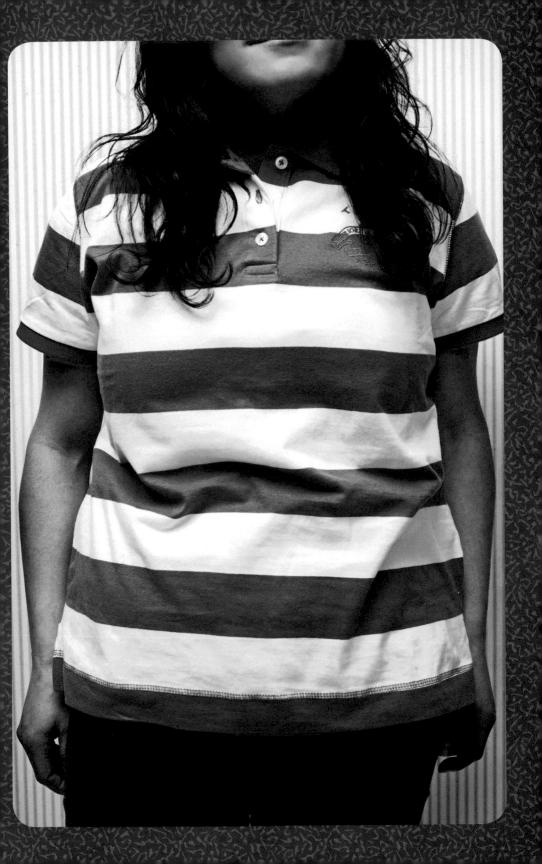

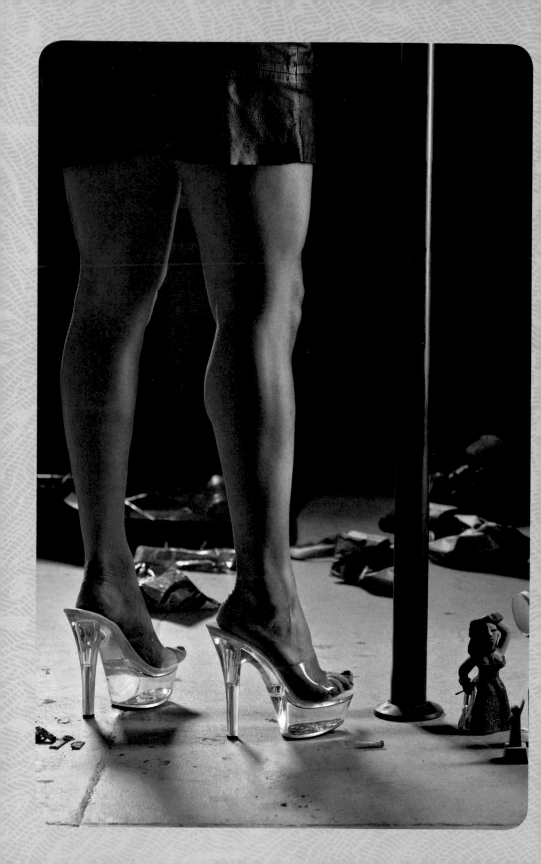

slut shoes

If you are a hooker or a stripper, I can understand why you might leave the house in a pair of platform Lucite stilettos. Marketing is marketing, and hey, a girl's gotta eat. But if your name is Jessica, and you work in a doctor's office five days a week, and you think it's fun to wear a skintight, strapless, black latex minidress and six-inch heels to Hound Dog Harry's on Saturday night for all-you-can-drink, two-dollar apple martinis, *you are a dumb slut*. Yes, Jessica, * I'm talking to you, *you dumb slut*. Those were seven-hundred-dollar Gucci loafers you ruined with apple martini vomit, but you wouldn't know that because you're, yes, a *dumb slut*.

* Names have been changed so dumb slut doesn't sue me for defamation of character! I would also like it known that I don't judge people based on the supposed looseness of their morals — just on their wardrobes.

gap in the back

The most common alteration I do for my clients, besides hemming pants and sleeves, is fixing Gap in the Back, a problem of which you are all too aware if you carry your weight in your hips and/or rump but have a relatively small waist. Yes, it's a drag when things don't fit perfectly off the rack, but that doesn't mean you should settle. People with great style don't settle! When I see a woman who has chosen to walk around with all that extra room in the back of her pants, I wonder why she doesn't make good use of it—you know, treat it as a marsupial-esque ass-pouch for storing her belongings, like a turkey sandwich and a romance novel.

Gap in the Back is really nothing to get yourself worked up about. When you find pants that fit you beautifully everywhere except in the waist, buy the damn things. Then find someone who knows how to sew. A small gap can be fixed with a little nip in the center of the waistband. A larger gap can be closed with two darts on the waistband, one over each butt cheek. When you get the pants back—*voilà*—they'll fit and you'll feel silly for whining about how pants never fit you.

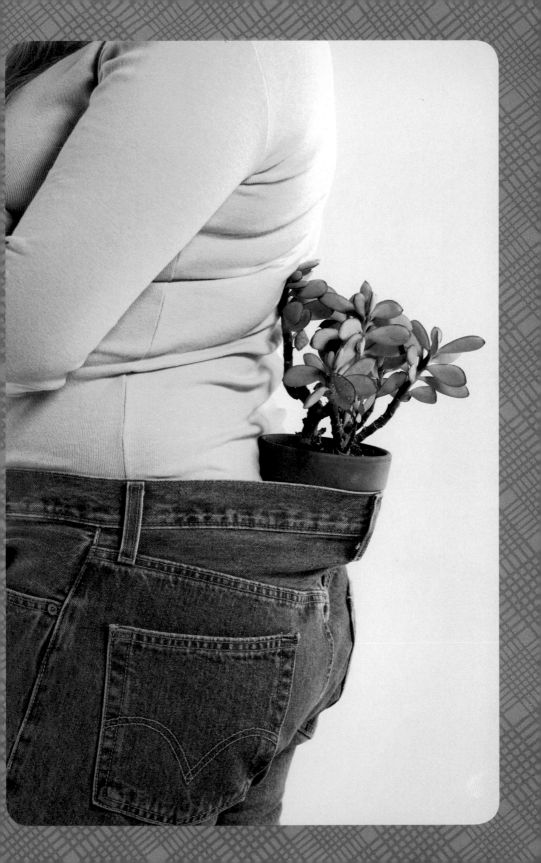

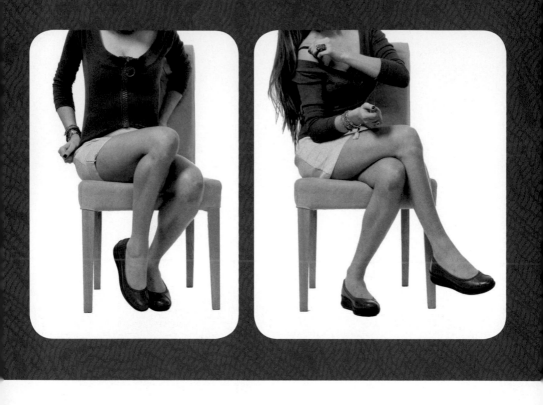

fidgeting

You can be wearing the cutest freakin' outfit in the whole world, but you'll look a helluva lot less beautiful if you spend half the night adjusting your bra straps and picking a wedgie out of your butt.

People with True Style:

1. Wear flattering clothes
2. Behave appropriately
3. Exude confidence

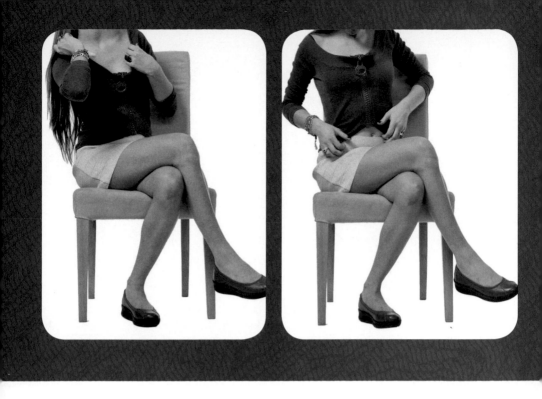

Fidgeting or fussing with a garment is a sign that something doesn't fit (that's strike number one) or that you don't have the confidence or composure to successfully pull off the look you're trying to achieve (strikes two and three).

If it's a question of fit, you *must* determine the reason the garment doesn't stay put—and fix it. Is your skirt riding up your thighs? It's probably too tight. Maybe it can be let out. If not, you need to let it go. Does your strapless dress keep sliding down the boobies? Well, if you have to hoist it up every two minutes, the bodice is too loose! So have it taken in. Or, here's a brilliant idea, wear a dress with straps next time. Whatever the reason, figure it out and do something about it.

If you're fidgeting due to a lack of confidence, it might be because you haven't found your true style just yet. But I'll give you a piece of advice: Confidence can be faked. Just take a deep breath, relax, smile, and be in the moment. Before long, you won't have to fake it anymore. Or you can just take a beta-blocker. Your choice.

giveaway and sloganed t-shirts

You walked a 5K. Congratu-freakin'-lations. How about you just *tell* people you strolled the whopping 3.125 miles instead of wearing the free, one-size-fits-all cotton tee they gave you at the finish line.

You attended a huge family reunion and your third cousin-in-law made a commemorative shirt. News flash: Nobody gives a rat's ass.

Your parents went to Aruba and all you got was this lousy T-shirt. That is so funny. Tell your parents you're going to wear that shirt the day you check them into the nursing home.

Whether you were given a T-shirt or had a momentary brain fart and bought one, I urge you to really think about: *a.* what it's doing for your body—probably nothing good—and, *b.* what it says about you—probably that you don't have one original thought rattling around in that brain of yours.

Are there funny statement tees in the world? Sure. Are there well-made ones? Yeah. Are there well-fitting ones? You betcha. But the vast majority—we're talking 99.99 percent of all sloganed or giveaway T-shirts—are lame-o, unflattering, and of poor quality.

Oh, one more thing: If you think it's funny to walk around in public wearing a T-shirt detailing the twenty-seven ways you can use the F-word, you are a loser and should be sterilized.

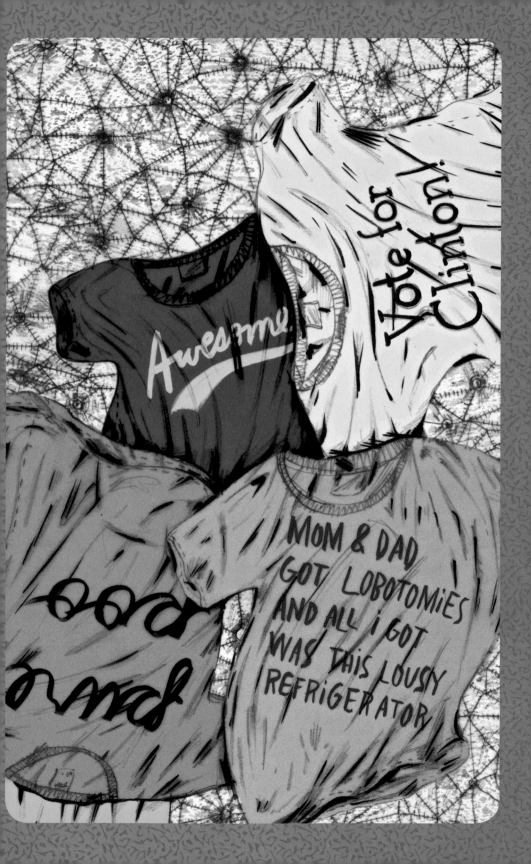

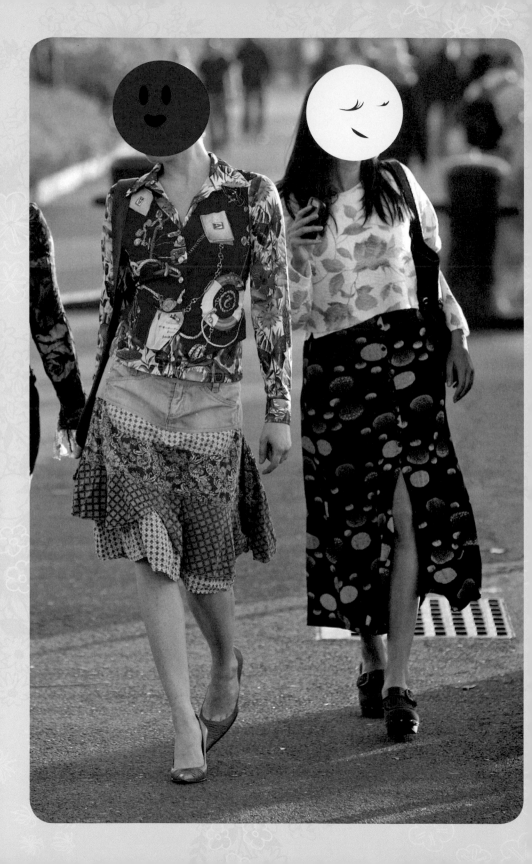

outdated patterns

If you were house hunting and you found one with an avocado green refrigerator, a pink toilet, and a bunch of brass trim, you'd probably laugh about it later with friends. Well, I do the same thing when I see a woman wearing chintz, except I don't wait until later. It's like Tourette's—I can't help it.

Outdated patterns make you look out of touch with society and can age you at least a decade. Of course, retro patterns often become trendy, but they're usually done in modern cuts and in modern fabrics. More often, over the course of any given decade or so, prints will develop a general feeling to them. For example, in the recent past, florals have trended away from looking like literal renditions of flowers and moved toward the abstract. *
And painterly prints have been gaining popularity.

To look modern you have to shop on a regular basis in trendy stores and occasionally pick up a magazine to see what fashionable people are wearing!

* As this book was going to press, little pink & purple rosebud florals (à la "Little House on the Prairie") became all the rage. Who can keep up with this crap?! You can!

double bubble
(or, thy cups runneth over)

The next time you want to give a man a piece of your mind for staring at your boobs, make sure the reason he's looking at your rack is not that he's wondering why you have four breasts instead of two. Double bubble occurs when a woman with a decent-size chest wears a bra that is too small, and then tops it off with a clingy knit. Disaster!

Ladies, ladies, ladies. How many times do I have to tell you this? You must have a professional bra fitting every two years, even if your weight has remained constant, or anytime you gain or lose a minimum of ten pounds. I can almost guarantee that after a professional bra fitter gets her hands on your bingo-bongos, you will discover that you are bigger in the cup and smaller in the band than you had previously thought. I know this because I have performed approximately one thousand booby makeovers in the past seven years. (See Low Boobies, page 23.)

And don't confuse lingerie with supportive undergarments. The same bra you wear in the bedroom to get your partner's blood flowing is not the same bra you wear to work.

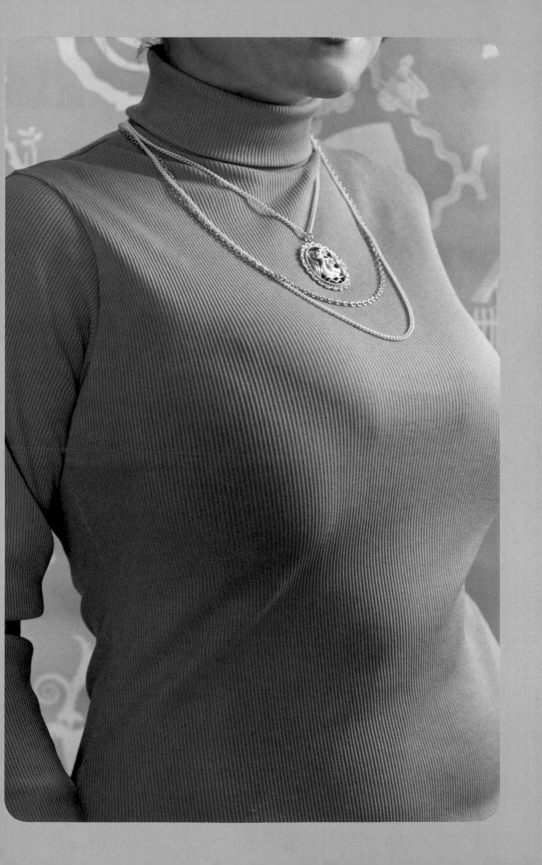

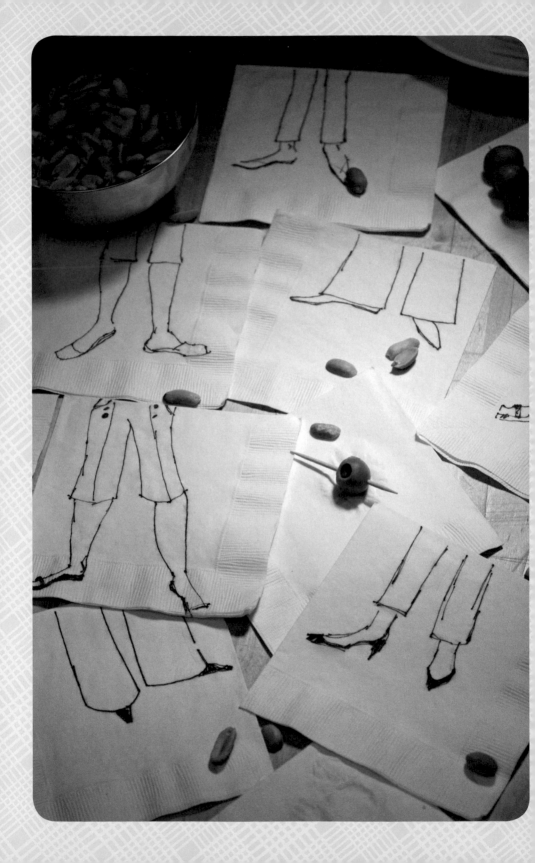

cropped pants

Women ask me constantly, "What do you have against cropped pants?" The truth is, I'm kind of fine with cropped pants—when they look good. But they rarely do. I am beyond-a-shadow-of-a-doubt convinced that the vast majority of women buy them because their length is one less thing to worry about. "Well, they fit in the waist! It doesn't matter what *length* they are." That makes about as much sense as Carrot Top's new face.

You can't just go around wearing pants any length you want! It doesn't work that way. Try to achieve one of the following lengths, or your look will have that neither-here-nor-there quality I find so damn annoying.

- Full-length pants should rest about a half an inch off the floor in the back.
- Full-length jeans should rest about a quarter of an inch off the floor in the back.
- Skinny jeans should hit at the ankle or be worn stacked (pushed up).
- Pedal pushers should hit just below the kneecap.
- Walking shorts hit just above the kneecap.
- Clamdiggers are meant to hit at midcalf.
- Ankle pants should be cropped just above the ankle bone.

The shorter and wider you are, the more likely you are to look like Spanky from the "Little Rascals" in a cropped pant. Wear Bermuda shorts or long pants instead!

porn mouth

Look, if you've gotta pay the bills by f#$^&*# complete strangers and simultaneously s%$#@&^ three c#@!$ on camera, I guess you have an excuse for outlining your mouth with dark lip liner and filling in the rest with frosty pink gloss. The rest of you, cut the $@*#. It makes you look like a slut.

I asked Carmindy what she thinks of DMS (dirty mouth syndrome), and let me tell you, she's not a fan. In fact, she says colored lip liner is an abomination. "It's ridiculously outdated," she says. Why do women still do it? I asked. "To give the illusion of fuller lips. But a much better trick is to use a clear highlight pencil and trace around the perimeter of your mouth," says Carmindy.

And what about that frosty stuff?

"Really glittery frost is old-school—and not in a good way," she says. She recommends modern pearlescent shimmer. When in doubt, put a little on your wrist and hold it up to the light. If you see actual flecks of mica, leave that goo at the makeup counter. Instead it should be shimmery, like oil on water.

Thanks, Carms. You're a doll.

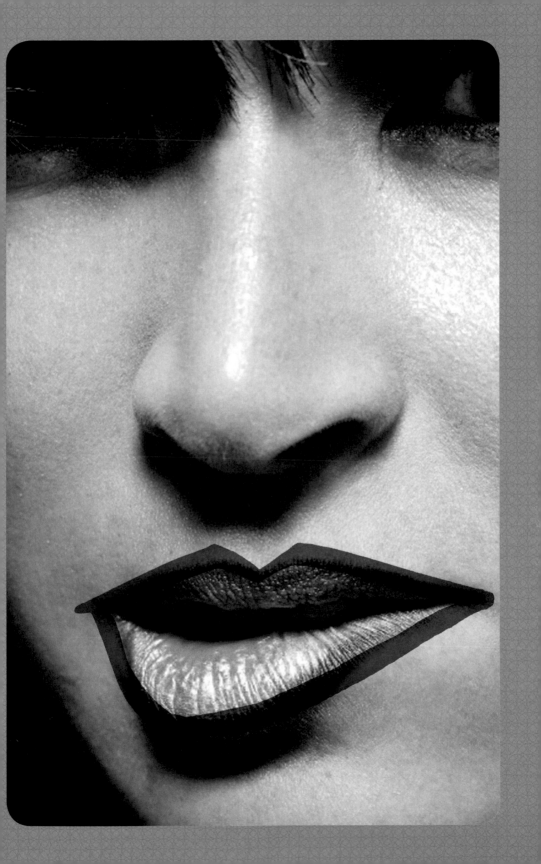

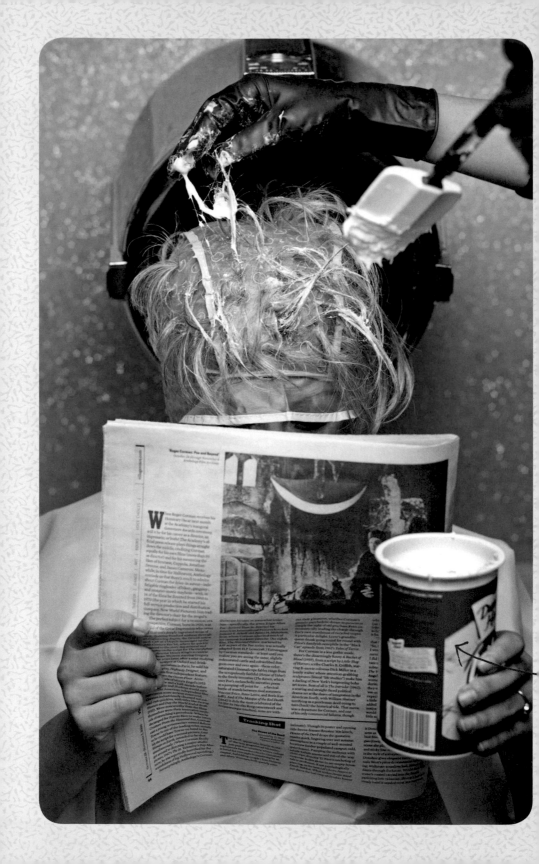

frosted hair

When I was a kid, about eight or so, I walked into my friend Pete's house while his mother was frosting her hair. I remember it like it was yesterday. She was talking on her yellow, corded rotary phone, while smoking a Pall Mall and stirring a pot of chili. On her head she wore this perforated cap with pieces of hair pulled through that were all sticking up like that scary dude from *Hellraiser*. I was supposed to spend the night, but I got really scared that Pete's mom might kill me in my sleep, so I ran home and told my mother I had diarrhea. When you say you have diarrhea, your mom is sympathetic but not overly concerned. It was the perfect ruse.

The next day I went to Pete's house to play kickball. His mom had all these white stripes in her hair that I couldn't stop staring at. She must have noticed because she asked, "Do you like my hair, Clint?" I said it was pretty. She thanked me and offered me some Kool-Aid. I was a convincing liar even before puberty.

Frosted hair went out of style right about the time Whitesnake did. Frosting has been replaced by highlights and lowlights. (If your "highlights" look like all the color has been stripped out of your hair in a clumsy assemblage of racing stripes, they qualify as "frosted.") Highlights are supposed to add brightness, not make your hair look damaged and dead. This is especially important as you age, when your skin loses some of its natural luster. Brightening your hair is an easy way to add vivacity to your overall appearance. Lowlights add more saturated color and depth to your hair—also a great way to make your hair appear healthier and more modern.

get it? that's cake frosting.

visible panty line

For some reason, VPL is one of my least favorite acronyms. It could be because I did an interview with some two-bit radio personality about six years ago and he just went on and on about VPL, VPL, VPL. I thought, *If this turd thinks the term VPL is cool, it must be incredibly uncool.* It's like when someone over the age of eighteen says things like "totes adorbs." Painful.

Nevertheless, visible panty line is a senseless style crime. Its crime-crime equivalent would be something like, oh, I don't know . . . breaking into someone's house and replacing their tacky wedding photo with an equally tacky oil portrait of a sad clown. Senseless. Don't let it happen to you.

The bigger and bulkier your panties, the more likely you are to get caught with a case of VPL. So if you're wearing light-colored or clingy trousers, try a thong or seamless shapewear.

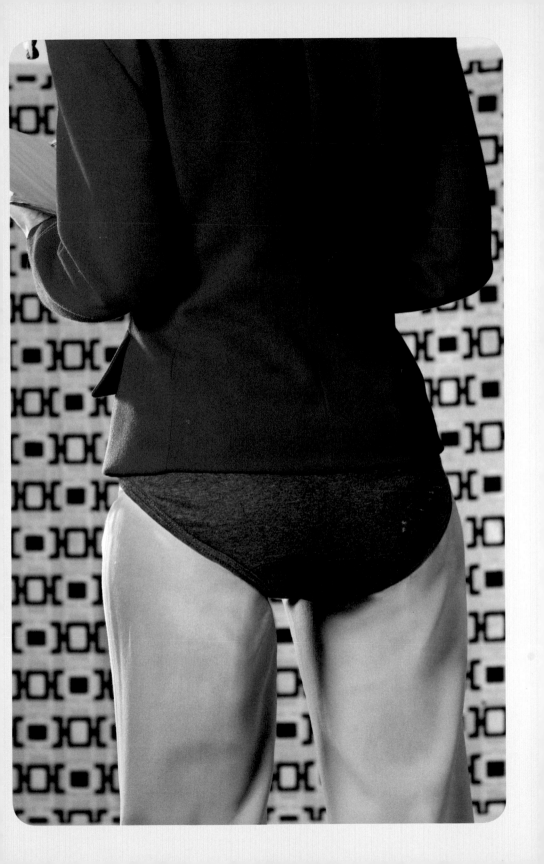

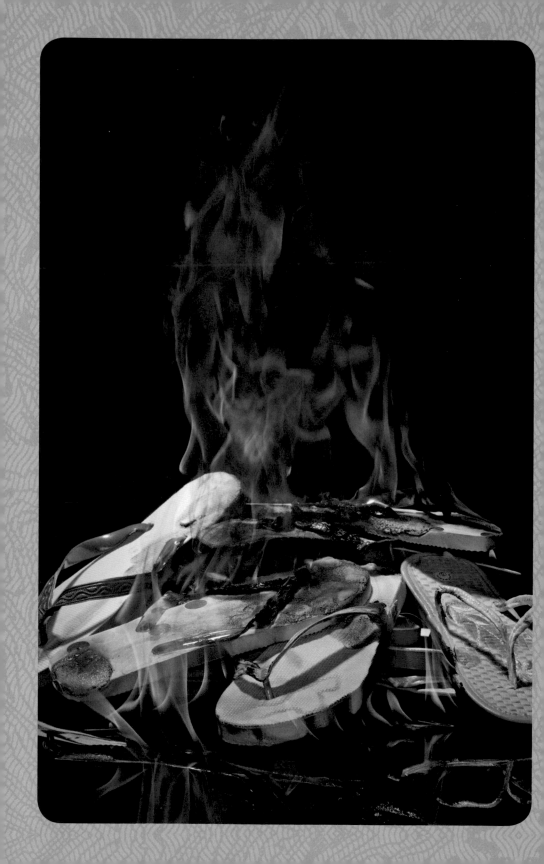

flip-flops

I will be honest. I love my flip-flops. But I'm also smart enough to know that there are times you shouldn't wear them. Granted, I'm not as smart as Judge Judy, because she's the smartest person on the planet. But still, I'm no idiot. (And I'm not kidding about Judge Judy. I sometimes fantasize that I am in her courtroom and I convince her, using my powers of logic and deference, that I have been wronged. Then she awards me the maximum five thousand dollars. Oh, my God, if that ever happened I would probably jump up and down like a spastic schoolgirl who forgot her Ritalin.)

Flip-flops are meant for the beach or the pool. Sometimes you can run an errand in them. But don't wear them to work. Don't wear them to the dentist. Don't wear them to any special occasion. And don't wear them on an airplane, because if there's an emergency, you will be really sorry.

This may all seem like common sense, but evidently a lot of people are stupid. Plus, I've read that flip-flops aren't good for your tootsies because your toes have to point down when you walk (to keep the flip-flop from flying off), which isn't natural. Don't believe me? Look it up on "the computer thing." (That's what Judge Judy calls "a computer.")

midsection cling

Look, I get it. Many people carry their weight in their mid-sections. But anything that appears to have been vacuum-sealed to your waist should be avoided at all costs, to avoid making you look like a stuffed sausage.

The number one way to draw attention away from your tummy is with a well-tailored jacket. Jackets strengthen the shoulder and create a strong vertical line up the front of the body. Many are also designed to narrow at the lower rib cage and flare away at the hip, creating an hourglass silhouette even if you don't have one.

Many women think that jackets are too fancy. I would argue that a denim, corduroy, or cotton blazer is indeed fancier than a hoodie, but certainly not too fancy for life in modern America. Other women say, "It's too hot to wear jackets here in _____!" (Insert southern Florida, Palm Springs, or San Antonio.) Maybe it's just me, but every time I'm in Florida, I end up freezing my ass off because the AC is cranked down to forty-two degrees everywhere I go. But whatever. If it is too hot to wear a jacket, look for blouses with some sort of detail under the bust, which adds extra fabric in the tummy. The empire seam is the most common of these details.

Oh, yes, here it comes: "But I feel like I'm wearing a maternity top!" And yes, it is true: If your tummy is bigger than your bust, you will look pregnant in an empire-waist blouse. Those work best in concealing a smaller pouch. Look for an empire band instead, something an inch or more in thickness, which will diminish the bun-in-the-oven appearance. I often tell women to look for a top that looks like there's a simple A-line skirt under the bust.

Other tricks include a knot under the bust or a little crisscross. Sometimes a little elastic smocking or an obi-like sash can camouflage a tummy. But what does *not* hide a tummy is any shirt that looks like a rectangle when you hold it up.

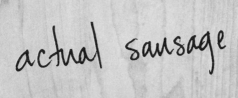

good brows ⟶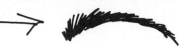

Bad brows ↓

slutty brow

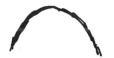

dude brow

trailer brow

invisible brow

bad brows!

Not too many people know this about me, but when I'm bored I draw women's eyebrows. Not on actual women, although I do think I would enjoy that. I do it on paper. I'm kind of obsessed with eyebrows, actually. Perhaps one day I will throw in the towel and open a little threading shop on Sixth Avenue and Fourteenth Street. Just kidding. I hate that corner. It smells like ass.

I'm not sure if I can adequately express to you just how important a well-shaped brow is to your entire face. Basically, that linear assortment of hairs above your eyes dictates how the rest of your mug will be judged. A smartly sculpted brow can enhance your bone structure, make your eyes look bigger, and give you an air of being better than everyone else. On the flip side, the wrong eyebrow can make you look crazy, low-class, Greek, or like a dude. Worst-case scenario is that you look like a crazy low-class Greek dude, which is cool, I guess, if you live above your parents' restaurant and grow a five-o'clock shadow on your back.

I'm digressing. Probably because I'm drunk. But not too drunk to explain the basic equation for shaping your brows.

1. Look at your face in the mirror.
2. Locate your tear duct.

3. Align a straight object, preferably an eyebrow pencil, vertically from your tear duct to your brow. This is where your brow should begin. We'll call it Point A.

4. Now keep one end of the pencil next to your nose and angle it so that it passes just to the other side of your pupil. Where the pencil meets your brow is where it should arch, in other words, its highest point. That's Point B.

5. Align the pencil with the outside corner of your eye. Follow the line up to your brow. This is where your brow should end. This is Point C.

6. One at a time, remove hairs, if necessary, to create a graceful arch that tapers gently from Point B to Point C. Take many breaks to step away from the mirror to make sure you haven't gone pluck-happy.

7. Repeat on other side.

Or . . . have a professional do it, which I highly recommend. The best way to approach this is to find an eyebrow expert in your area through word of mouth. She might use wax or thread or tweezers. Doesn't matter much—except if you have very delicate skin, in which case wax might not be your best option.

You don't have to pay a hundred bucks every week or anything, just have those bushy babes shaped once and maintain them yourself at home. With a good pair of tweezers, remove the new growth, one hair at a time.

P.S. I love greek people!

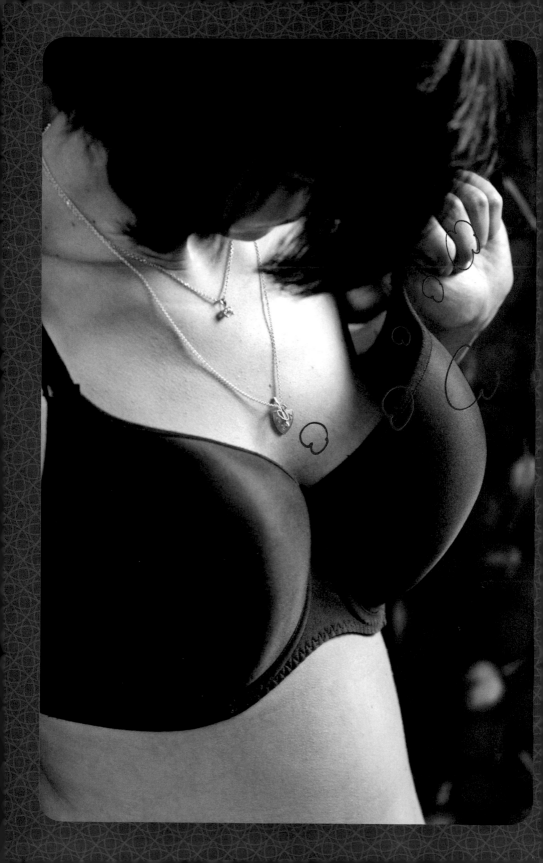

underfilled cups

God bless the foam-cup bra, for it gives the smaller girls some added oomph. But beware: A foam demi-cup when not filled to capacity makes your ta-tas seem tiny. I don't usually consider myself a pessimist, but it's hard to see the cup as half full when it's really half empty.

Solution: If you have a small chest, a professional bra fitting is just as important as it is for bustier babes (see Double Bubble, page 92). The breast should fill the cup of the bra, plain and simple. There's no leaving extra room for your hopes and dreams.

pastel pink

Sometimes it's fine to wear pastel pink. Those times would be if: Your name is Rose Nylund and you hail from St. Olaf, Minnesota.✱ You are a girl who has not yet had her first monthly visitor. You are Molly Ringwald and it is 1985. You are an Easter egg.

Super-pale pink can be very chic in say, a chiffon blouse, if you have beautiful skin (see Beige, page 76), but in general, pastel pink tends to look very dated, specifically back to the 1980s, its heyday. Unfortunately, pastel pink "evolved" into dusty rose in the early '90s, and everyone had to have it in their kitchens and bathrooms. Then the whole country overdosed on it and moved on to granite, which should look dated any minute now.

If you're going to wear pastel pink, make certain that it's done in a very modern style (maybe a skintight backless sheath with a really bold zipper detail or an asymmetric silk blouse). Generic apparel such as turtlenecks, cardigans, and jackets done in pastel pink will automatically age you at least a decade. Add a strand of pearls and you've added another ten years. And a special note to my ladies "over a certain age," more saturated colors look best on older skin because, as we age, we lose some coloring. You can brighten your appearance with brighter and/or richer colors—in general, you should veer toward jewel tones. And if you love pink so much, try fuchsia, which is a much easier color to wear.

✱ Only "Golden Girls" reference in book.

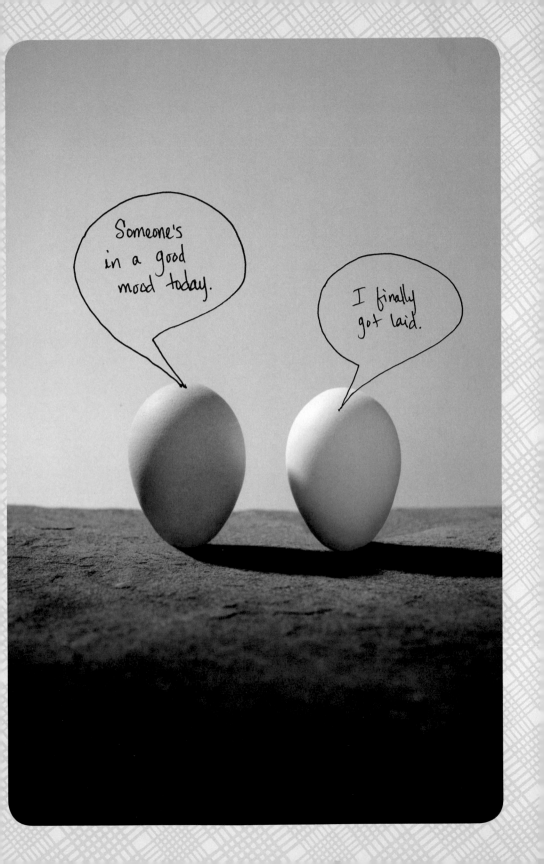

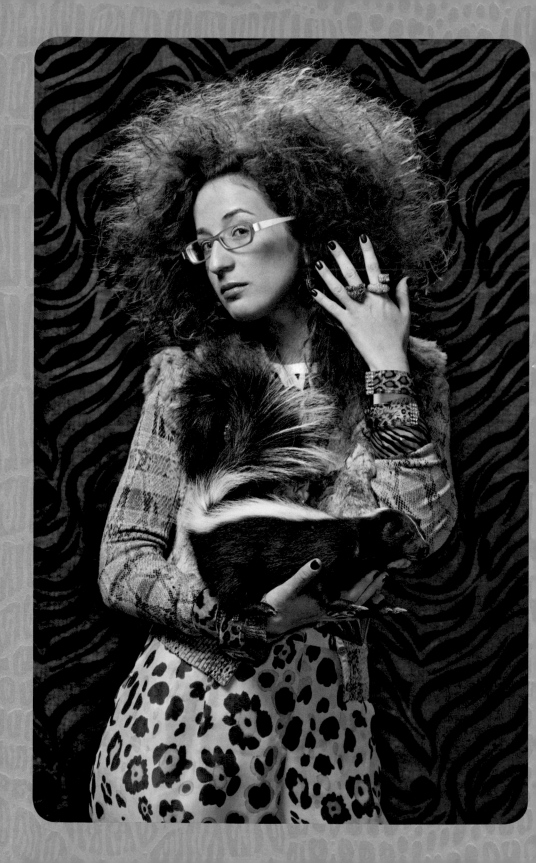

attacked by animal print

I love a woman who loves animal print because, just by looking at her, I can tell she's not a shrinking violet. Animal print wearers, based on my vast experience, have strong opinions, enjoy their femininity, and usually like to have a good time. Women who wear *too much* animal print, however, usually have strong opinions about things that don't make any sense, enjoy the company of longshoremen, and drink too much blackberry brandy. And wear too much damn perfume.

First and foremost, animal print should fit close to the body. Loose-fitting animal print makes you look like you just killed and skinned a beast, like Jane of the Jungle.

Once you find pieces that fit, wear them one at a time. Animals that don't hang out together in nature won't coexist peacefully on your body either. Wear a leopard-print pencil skirt with a brown silk blouse and burgundy heels. Wear a zebra-print cardigan with jeans and cute flats. Wear python pumps with a little black dress. Don't wear the leopard-print pencil skirt, zebra cardigan, and python shoes all at once. You'll look like a freak from *The Island of Doctor Moreau*. (Crappy movie. Don't even bother renting it.)

I also think animal print should be worn in moderation, about once every two weeks (shoes being exempt from this rule). I'm all for a trademark look, but being known as the animal print lady is just one step away from becoming a crazy cat lady. No one takes you seriously, and everyone avoids your calls.

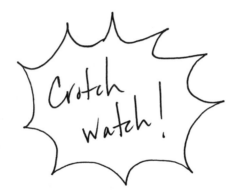

camel toe

I'm not going to beat around the bush here. If others can see your labia majora while you are fully clothed, your pants are too tight. I don't care how much you love them, they no longer fit and there's no use pretending they do. It's time to give up the ghost and send those dromedaries packing. Donate them to the charity of your choice for someone two sizes smaller to wear and spread the love.

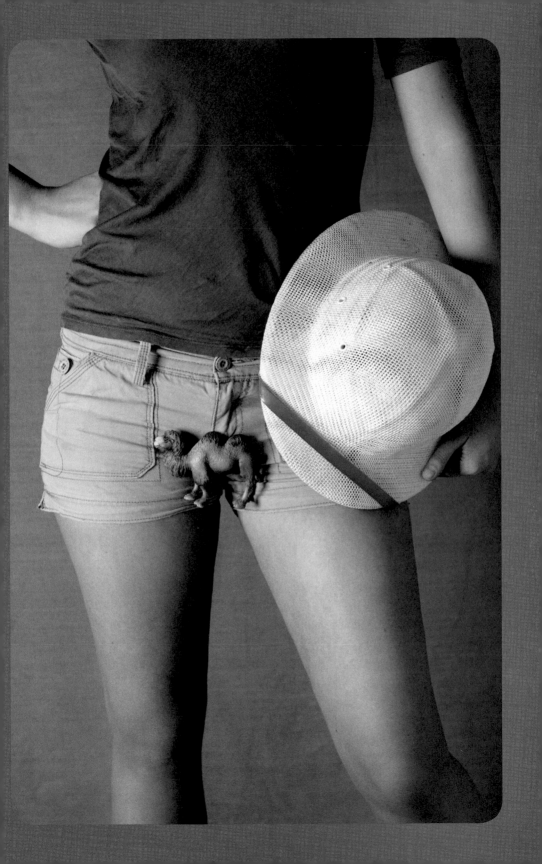

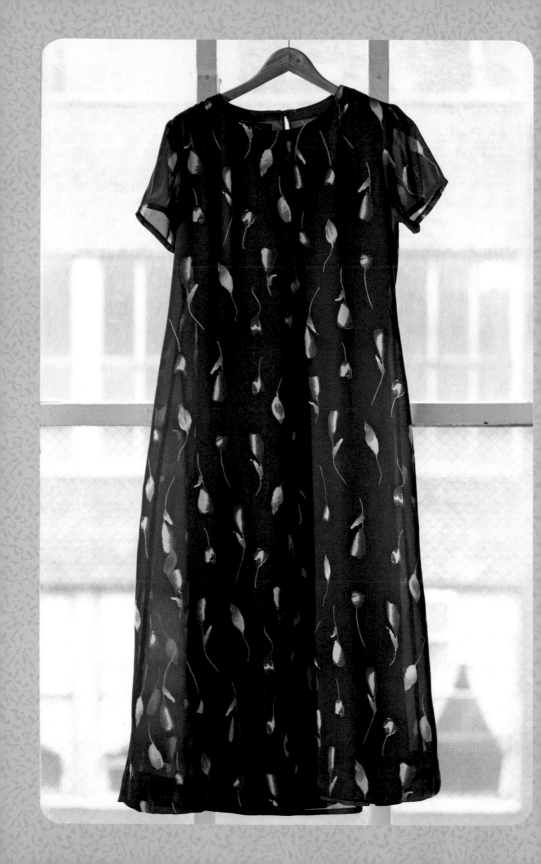

the "i give up" dress

"I have a wedding to go to this weekend, so I went to the mall and tried on three dresses and nothing really fit perfectly—I have a tricky body type—so when I saw this hanging on the rack, I figured, what the hell, I'll try it on. I mean, it's gotta fit; it's really just two curtains sewn together at the top and sides, with holes for the arms and head. And the print is so pretty—great big pink, larger-than-life roses on a yellow background, always a classic. It hits just above the ankle, which is what I think they call tea length. I'll wear it with a sensible shoe and the fake pearls Grandma left me in her will and sort of sit off to the side."

This sad excuse for a dress ranks up there with the Mom Jean (page 2) and white Cross-trainers (page 67) as one of the greatest style tragedies ever to befall the American woman. I beseech you to destroy any rectangular, floral frock in your closet that hangs limply on your body with zero waist definition. YOU CANNOT WEAR IT JUST BECAUSE IT IS SOLD IN STORES AND BECAUSE A MILLION OTHER WOMEN HAVE BOUGHT IT.

Ladies, you must, must, must define a waist. The essence of the female silhoutte is the hourglass. If you hold a garment up on the hanger and it is shaped like a child's building block, it will not be flattering on you, especially if you have any curves whatsoever. (Women built like coatracks have an easier time wearing boxy dresses, and even then I'd probably recommend a belt.)

Yes, a woman who is five foot six and a perfectly proportioned size 6 will have an easier time finding cocktail dresses. Such is life. That does not mean the rest of you can give up and wear window treatments. Look for dresses that have shape built into them and let the dress do the work for you. Here's a formula that I find works 99 percent of the time. If you can find one dress with these three criteria, you should be golden:

1. **V-NECK** (works on large chests and smaller ones)

2. **A HIGH, DEFINED WAIST**
   (almost a cummerbund under the bustline)

3. **A FLARED SKIRT** to the knee

Say it with me : V-neck, defined waist, flared skirt.

Write it down on your hand if you have to and get thyself to the mall!

dated hair

I am regularly amazed—and I mean amazed—by the number of women across this country sporting hairstyles that were popular twenty years ago or that are just plain crappy. I really don't understand it.

Once and for all, this is how you get a good haircut: Find someone who has a cute hairstyle, who is roughly your age, and who has a similar hair texture to yours. Then you approach her and ASK HER WHO CUTS HER HAIR!

If you live in Pittsburgh, this could take years, so you can always visit a newsstand. I'm not a big fan of tabloid magazines (because I don't give a rat's ass about Heidi, Spencer, or their general ilk), but the rags are a pretty easy way to keep in touch with modern hair. Look for a celebrity who's your age, has your coloring, and is pretty. Granted, tabloids usually don't write about women over forty, but look through other mags. Rip out the page and take it to the salon. Say, "I'd like this, please. And if you get it right I will tip you generously."

Why do I have to tell you this? I've gotten all worked up and I've insulted Pittsburgh, a beautiful city (really) that doesn't deserve my scorn. Look what you make me do.

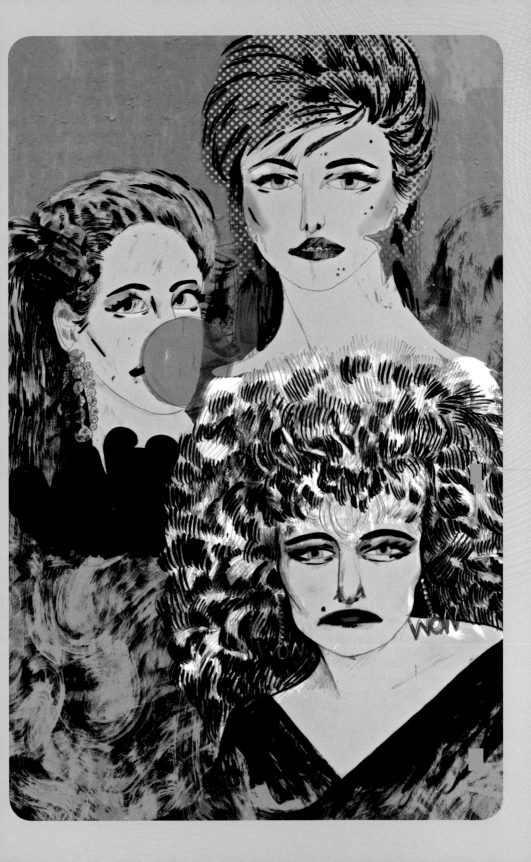

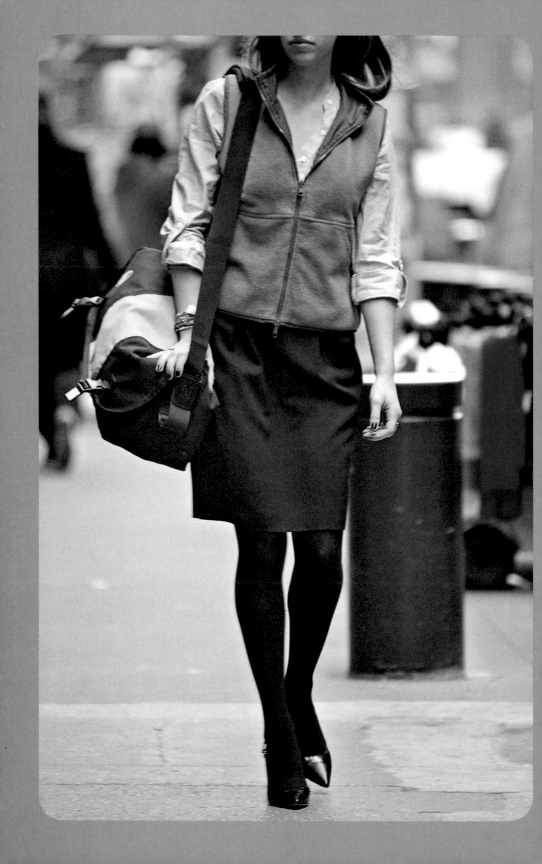

polar fleece

This is a map of the United States.

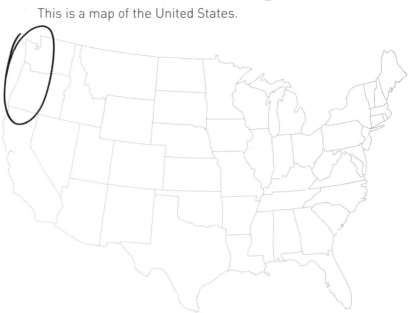

The parts I have circled are experiencing an epidemic: polar fleece addiction. That's right, Pacific Northwest, I'm talking to you! What are you gonna do about it?

Polar fleece is great for a hike in the woods or walking the dog. It should not be worn to the office or in any restaurant that doesn't serve mozzarella sticks. Instead of a fleece pullover, go get yourself a jacket. Maybe something in cotton canvas, corduroy, denim, tweed, wool, leather, linen, silk . . . the list goes on.

"But it's cool and rainy!" you say.

Hmmmm . . . if only someone would invent a garment specifically designed for wet weather that is both insanely chic and quite comfortable. It would be about knee-length and roomy enough to fit over another jacket or other layering piece, such as a sweater. Maybe it would belt at the waist. It could come in a variety of fabrics and finishes, with tan being the most popular.

Oh, wait, someone already did that, like a hundred years ago. It's called a trench coat. You polar fleece addicts are really starting to piss me off.

any sort of belly-baring shirt when you have stretch marks

Ah, yes, the miracle of life. Babies are beautiful. Pregnant women are beautiful. I wish you and your child a lifetime of laughter, joy, and codependence. I also wish you would spare me from looking at the starfish around your belly button just because you feel sexy in a tube top and are on the lookout for another fine gentleman to impregnate you.

Get some freakin' class. And spare your kid the MILF jokes on the playground.

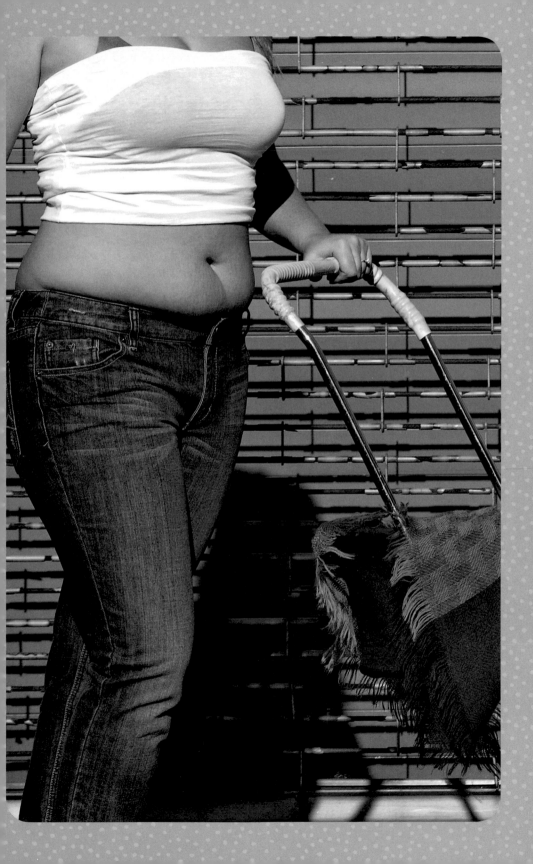

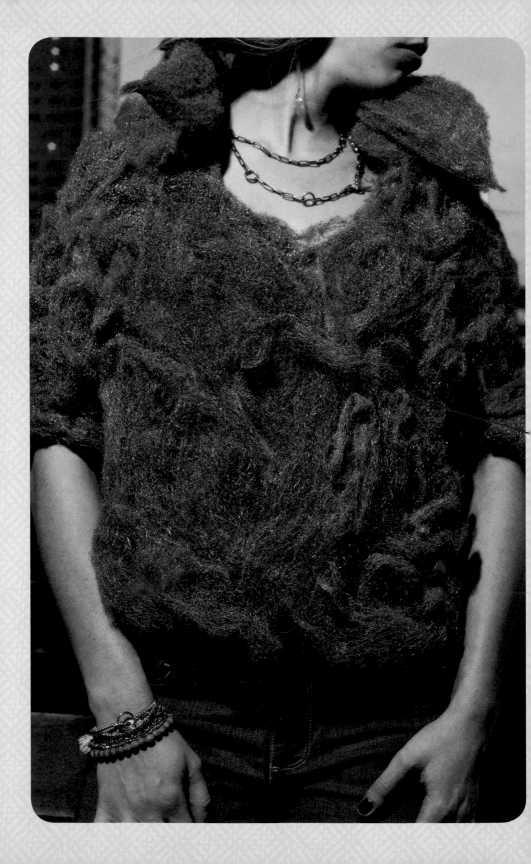

old-school polyester

All polyester is not evil; just the stuff that feels like a Scotch-Brite sponge. I have a general rule of thumb: If it can be used to scour a dishpan, remove chipped paint, or scrape Joan Collins's bunions, don't make a blouse out of it. I'm a real maverick like that.

But man-made fibers can be quite useful. Great advances in technology have made polyesters infinitely softer than their 1950s ancestors. Generally, man-made fibers wash well and don't fade.

I always say, "You can't go wrong with a blend!" (I do always say that, by the way. Not as often as "Bartender, I'll have another." But still, quite a bit.) Natural fibers allow superior breathability and synthetics hold up in the wash. So when you combine them, everyone's happy.

we made this jacket out of steel wool!

head-to-toe trend ho

Nothing says "I'm desperate to be perceived as cool" more than a woman who chases every trend that blows into town and copies the exact looks of Hollywood's latest It girl. It's especially sad if she's had a face-lift and deliberately dumps kitty litter into her hot tub so she can have the pool boy vacuum it out. You know who you are.

Trends are important (see Opting Out, page 200). They're an expression of who we are as a society. Would the '50s have been the same without poodle skirts? Would the '80s have been the same without shoulder pads? Would my high school experience have been the same if I hadn't worn acid-wash, pleated taper jeans and a mullet? No, no, and probably . . . because I was a dork.

I usually recommend that women set a style budget for themselves at the beginning of the year. Whether that budget is $500 or $5,000, here's how I recommend you spend it:

- If you are a professional woman working in a creative environment, or a nonworking woman under thirty-five-ish and financially solvent, spend 75 percent of your style budget on trends and 25 percent on classics.
- If you're a woman working in a corporate environment, or a nonworking woman over thirty-five-ish who is financially solvent, spend 50 percent of your budget on trends and 50 percent on classics.
- If you are a woman with a limited budget or are facing financial uncertainty, spend 25 percent of your budget on trends and 75 percent on classics.

I can see your eyes glazing over from here because I'm talking about economics, so let me make this simple. You should absolutely participate in trends, but without being a slave to them. Fashion is the clothing and accessories offered to you. Style is putting your own spin on those pieces.

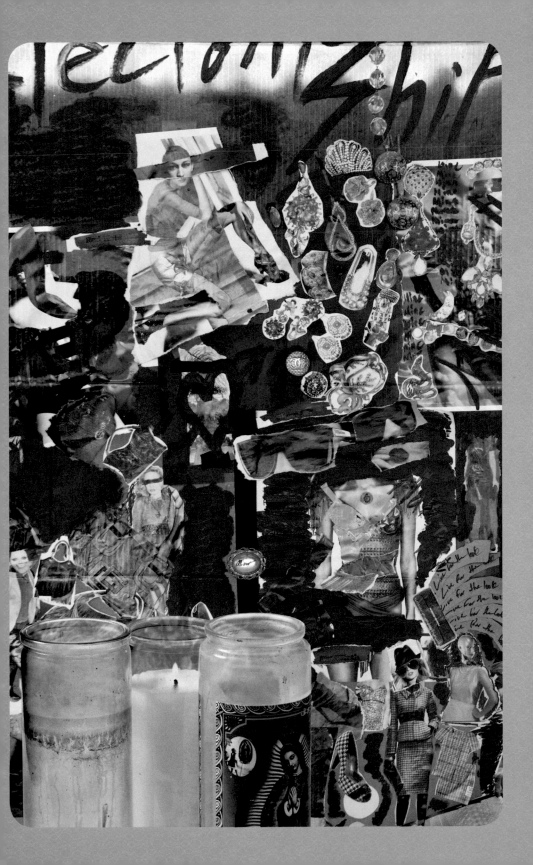

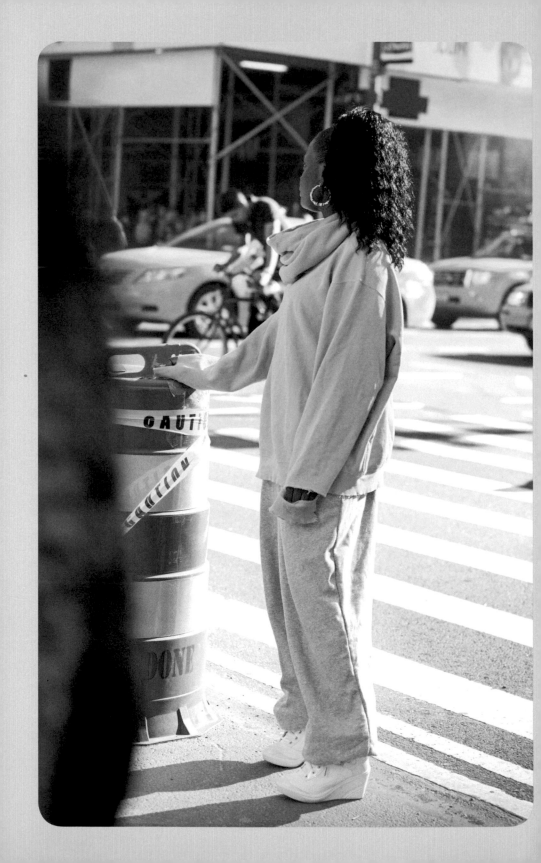

sweatshirts and their evil cousins, hoodies

No self-respecting woman over the age of twenty-two should ever leave the house in a sweatshirt, especially if she has no intention of sweating. I'll cut you a little slack if you're going to a football game or you live in a dorm, but even then you should know that inside, I am frowning upon you.

Why?

Because no one with even an ounce of good taste will look at you while you're wearing a sweatshirt and think, *Wow, that woman has a real sense of style,* or *Wow, that woman has a great body.*

Let's get this straight: Sweatshirts give the impression that you are slovenly and lazy. Perhaps even worse, they can make a beautiful figure look lumpier than a sack of dead cats—because they have absolutely no shape, no structure! I mean, look at the construction of a sweatshirt. It's a cloth bag with sleeves, and usually really wide, droopy sleeves at that. They're so uncomplicated you could probably teach a stoned monkey how to make one between bong hits.

Now, let's move on to the hoodie, which is basically a sweatshirt with a dangling, useless appendage 'round back. Who the hell let this look become so popular? I might enjoy the concept of the hoodie more if people actually utilized that pouch behind their necks. You could carry your cell phone in there. Or a bag of Cheetos. Or a premature baby . . . Now that I think about it, I *love* the idea! You could go to the mall, walk around for a few hours with your pack of underachiever friends, park your ass on a bench, dig around in your "clothes," then call your baby's daddy while eating cheese curls and nursing little Brit'ny. Ah, the American dream.

Look, hoodies are supercasual. Even cashmere ones can look a little sloppy. I know this because I own two of them. They're best relegated to housewear—wear them while dusting, watching the boob tube, cooking dinner for the young'uns. But think twice before you enter public spaces. You can tell yourself you look cute in a sweatshirt or a hoodie, but we both know you'd be lying.

mustaches

Recently, an acquaintance of mine was complaining that she was having a difficult time finding a boyfriend. She wondered if it could be her personality. I said I doubted it because she's pretty cool, maybe a little crazy, but so is everyone in New York. She said, "Maybe I need to work a little less." And I replied, "That's not it."

She said, "Well, what is it then?"

And I said, because I was drunk, "You've got hair on your upper lip. Guys don't like that. Most gay guys don't even like that on a man."

"But there are just a few," she exclaimed, "and I bleach them."

"Bleaching is not good enough," I replied. "Wax them, thread them, sugar them, electrocute them, do whatever it takes—but get those things off your face. Even if there are just three of them, it's three too many."

She was a little insulted, but she took my advice and now she has a boyfriend. He's a total loser, but at least she has someone to go to dinner with.

OMG!
Christina Aguilera!

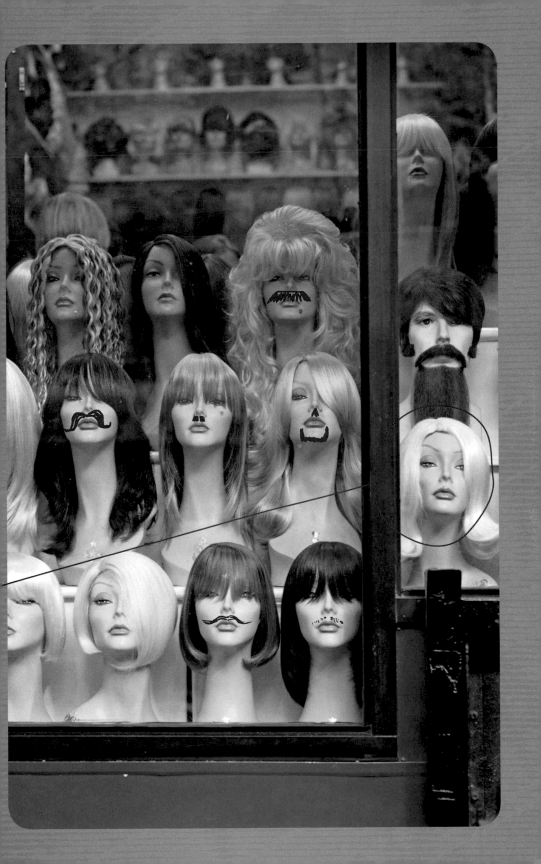

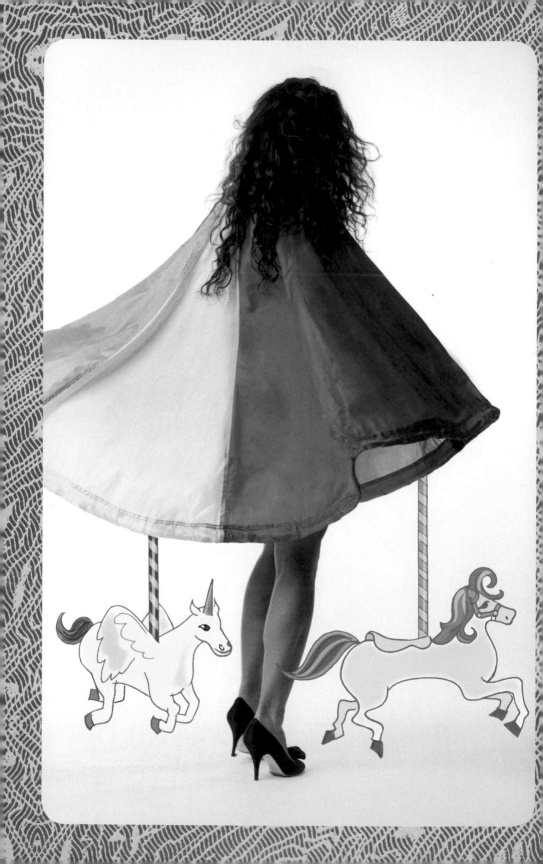

This one's for my bigger gals. Never, ever, let anyone tell you that because you're a plus size you need big, flowy tops and tent dresses to cover you up. That infuriates me! What you need is absolutely the opposite of loosey-goosey billowing fabric. You need structure, structure, structure. Sure, some designers would like you to believe that you need drapey stuff, because it's a hell of a lot easier to fit a poncho on a woman than it is a blouse. But do you really want to spend your life looking like one of the ghosts from Pac-Man?

If you don't have an hourglass shape, use clothes to give the illusion that you do. Is that easy? Absolutely not! The women's departments of many stores are limited to say the least, which means you'll have to try harder to find clothes that fit and flatter you. But I *beg* you not to give up.

The next time you're shopping, I want you to pay close attention to the construction of the clothes you're perusing. If it looks like a tent or a potato sack on the hanger, it's going to look the same on you. Look for seams. Seams create shape. Seams do the work so your body doesn't have to. Seams also give tailors opportunities for alterations.

And, if you are plus size and have any desire to have great style, you absolutely cannot do it without a great tailor. Do not, I repeat, do not feel defeated if a garment does not fit you perfectly off the rack. It is unreasonable for you to expect it to. One woman may be a size 16 because she has a large bust. Another might be a size 16 because she carries weight in her tummy. Yet another might be a size 16 because she has a broad back. How on earth is a designer supposed to fit every one of those women perfectly? It cannot be done.

Take my advice: Fit your biggest part and tailor down from there. If you have a tummy and you find a jacket you love, make sure it closes over the tummy, then take it to a tailor to alter the rest. That may mean resetting the shoulder, or narrowing the sleeve, or both. It will cost you some extra money, but in the end you will have a jacket that fits you perfectly, and good fit is the essence of good style.

droopy shoulders

The shoulder seam of a garment should sit on the outside edge of your shoulder. When it extends down your arm, you start to look slouchy and schlumpy. Women with very thin frames should pay particular attention to avoid droopy shoulders, because they can make you look scrawny. Last time I checked my thesaurus, *slouchy, schlumpy*, and *scrawny* were not synonyms for *stylish*. (Technically, *schlumpy* isn't even a word, but that's not important right now.)

What is important is noticing where shoulder seams hit on the body. A blouse doesn't necessarily fit just because you can get it over your head. If you have a larger frame and a relatively small shoulder, this will drive you crazy because, as I always say, you must go up in size until you fit your largest part and tailor the rest of the garment from there.

So what do you do if you have, say, a large bust and a small shoulder? Well, you must go up in size until you fit your bust. And if the garment is too big in the shoulder, you have the shoulder reset. Is that a complete and total pain in the rear? You betcha, but it has to be done. Sometimes I'll recommend small shoulder pads if a woman has a very narrow shoulder and a large bust or midsection. Within reason (read: not '80s style), they can help bring a little balance to the body.

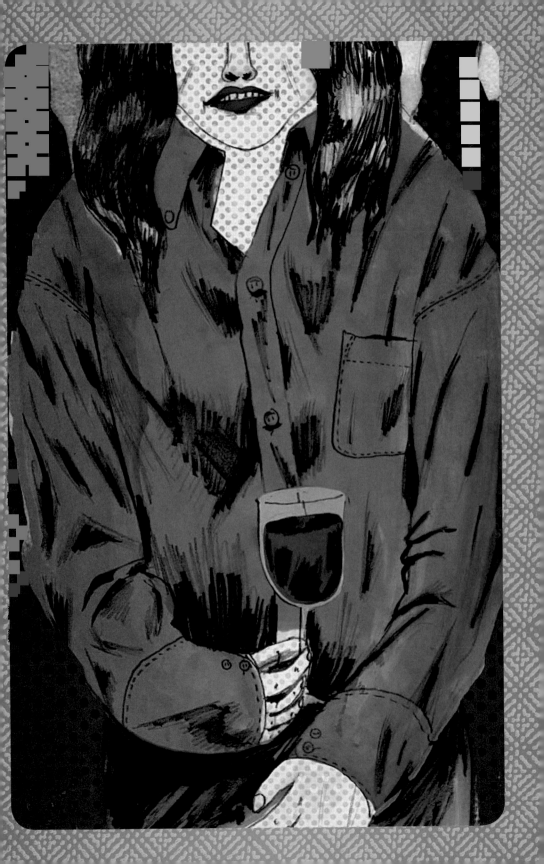

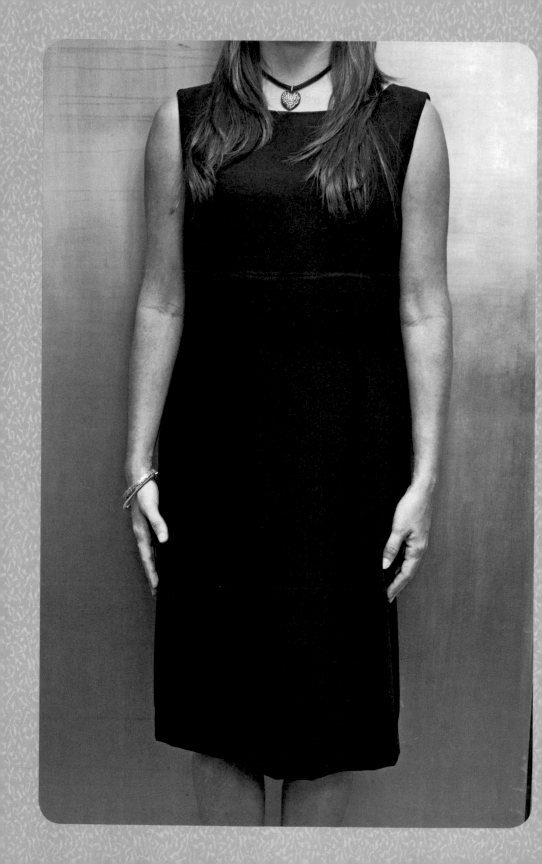

the LLBD
(lame little black dress)

Yes, yes, Coco Chanel did say every woman needs a little black dress, and I certainly don't disagree. But I'm pretty sure ole Coco would disapprove of your showing up at your cousin's wedding in a shapeless black sheath, mules, a leather bag on a long thin strap, and ¹⁄₁₆-carat diamond studs in your ears.

The point of the LBD is utility and cost effectiveness, not copping out. It should be the kind of garment you can dress down for day and up for evening. And it should be classic rather than trendy, so it will remain fashionable for years. In effect, it's a blank slate. And you can't wear a blank slate to a party. A canvas needs paint or it's just a canvas. The LBD needs accessories or it's just an LLBD.

In general, the more elaborate a garment is, the less ostentatious your accessories should be (unless you're attending a very fancy event). On the flip side, the simpler a garment, the more chances you can take with your jewelry, bag, and shoes.

The true test of an LBD is whether you can wear it with tights and a jacket for work, and also wear it to a cocktail party with strappy sandals, bold jewelry, and a clutch.

And when you find out where that cocktail party is, let me know. I'm jonesing for a G&T.

scrunchies
(and other cheap hair crap)

Seinfeld was a funny show. It stopped taping in 1998, after a successful nine-year run. During the final seasons, the character of Elaine, played by the beautiful and charming Julia Louis-Dreyfus, stopped wearing scrunchies on the top of her head—probably because she realized she looked like a freakin' idiot. They didn't even have cell phones back when *Seinfeld* aired, so we can chalk the rampant scrunchie abuse up to the naïveté of simpler times. But if you're still wearing a scrunchie now, wow, that is laaaaame.

If I were commissioner of the fashion police, the first law I would enforce is this one: Women, you are hereby allowed one scrunchie each, which under no circumstances is allowed to leave the bathroom. You may use the scrunchie only while removing your makeup, washing your face, or to tie your hair back while vomiting.

Keep in mind that everyone knows how much all those little drugstore-bought hair gizmos (butterfly clips, rhinestone barrettes, etc.) cost. They're like fifty-nine cents. You will never look "expensive" wearing a piece of crap like that on your head. If you're going to use an inexpensive hair doodad, buy an inconspicuous one, like a regular bobby pin or plain elastic. There's a general rule of thumb in style:

Hide the cheap.

Live it.

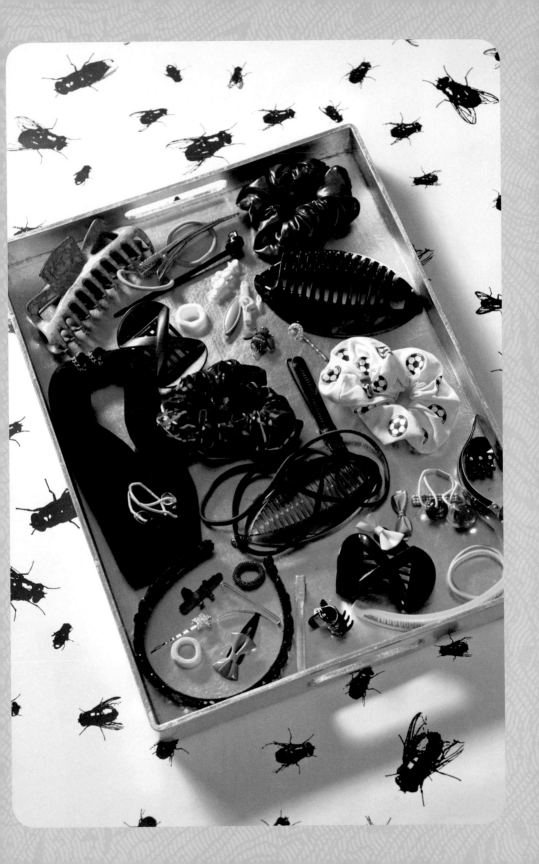

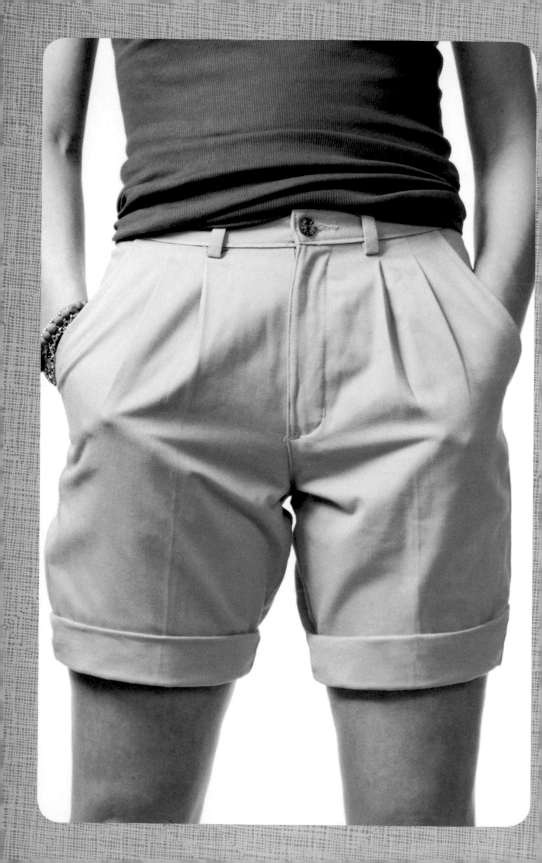

pleated khaki cuffed shorts

I admire lesbians. You're tough and you can fix things. Co-incidentally, these are some of the same qualities I love about my dad. However, I have noticed that many of you—and I'm not saying the majority, maybe 49 percent of you over the age of forty-five-ish—wear pleated khaki cuffed shorts in the summer. Don't tell me you don't. I've been to Provincetown, Key West, and Phoenix!

Do yourself a favor and eschew the gym teacher shorts in favor of walking shorts, also known as Bermuda shorts. They're a straight-leg short that hits at the top of the knee. For the cleanest, longest leg line possible, choose the un-cuffed version. And before you start experimenting with patterns, get yourself some nice solids, maybe black or navy blue if you've got really pale skin. And make sure they don't have pleats! Sheesh. Nobody likes a girl with a puffy crotch.

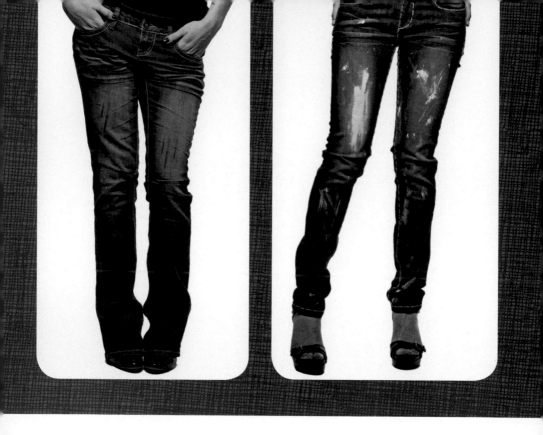

distressed denim

Jeans. They're as American as apple pie made with high-fructose corn syrup. Mmm-mmm. Unfortunately, not all jeans are so tasty.

Let's play a little game. I like to call it "logic." Answer A or B.

Your jeans are distressed, bleached, or faded on the thighs. They make your thighs look:
   A. thinner
   or
   B. thicker

Your jeans are distressed, bleached, or faded on the ass. They make your ass look:
   A. smaller
   or
   B. larger

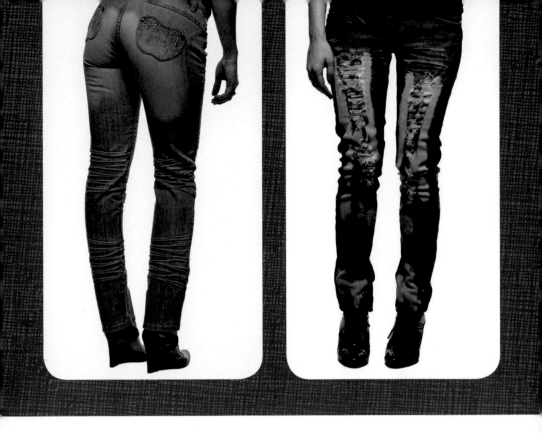

Your jeans are distressed, bleached, or whiskered on the hips. They make your hips look:

    A. narrower

    or

    B. wider

Okay, are you ready for the answers? Here goes . . . **B, B, B, B, B, B, B, B, BBBBBBBBBBBBBBBB!!!!!!!!!!!!!!!!!!!**

From now on, I want you to think of bleaching and/or fading as a magnifying glass for whatever's underneath it. If you've got *grande* thighs already, they'll look *mucho grande* when you put big white patches on them. In general, darker, uniform denim washes are more universally flattering. Also, rips and bleach stains are better left to teenagers, who can get away with looking like they don't give a crap. That's the beauty of being young; nobody expects you to look like a responsible adult. When you're fifty, however, and walking around looking like a skate punk, people, like me, think you're a loser.

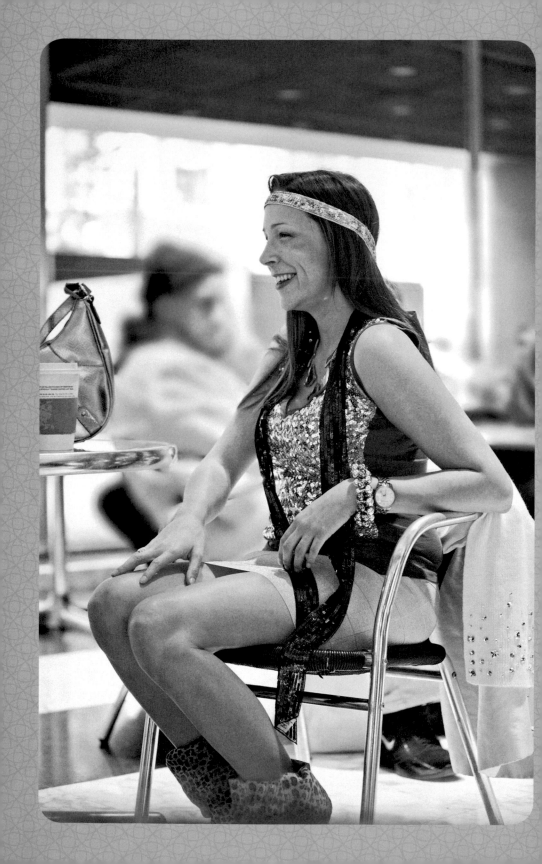

shine OD

Remember how I told you that four ingredients make a woman's outfit interesting—color, texture, pattern, and shine? (Technically, I haven't told you that yet. See "All Solids All the Time," page 166.) And I'm sure you've heard me say on TV that there's nothing wrong with a little shine for daytime. Well, I still stand behind all that, but I need to emphasize a concept called moderation.

Do not, I repeat, do not combine metallic shoes, bedazzled jeans, a sequined top, a jewel-embellished cardigan, and Mr. T's gold necklaces in the same outfit. I don't care if it's nuclear winter and those are the only clothes you own. You'll look like a crazy lady.

A little shine is great for day, but you need just a touch of it to make an impact. Choose ONE shiny garment, perhaps a sweater with a little Lurex thread in the knit, and add ONE shiny accessory.

For night, different rules apply. You can do shine or sheen from head to toe if the occasion calls for it. It will be best, however, if you keep the look focused. By that I mean don't mix too many kinds of shine. A red sequined dress is great. It might look great with some gold shoes and some diamond earrings. But it probably doesn't need a rhinestone clutch and a metallic shawl.

Nobody likes a burned retina.

"it's vintage!"

Overheard at a coffee shop: Twentysomething woman on her cell phone. She is wearing red lipstick and her bangs are rolled. She has obviously slept with pink foam curlers in her hair. "Holy crap. You are not going to believe this. I found the most amazing Mary Janes in a garbage can behind that old folks' home by the airport. They look like they were made in 1925 and have been resoled, like, fifty-seven times. I mean, I can only assume. Oh, and remember my aunt Frieda? Well, she died yesterday. No, it's cool, she was, like, ninety-three or something. When my mother told me she croaked, I went into her closet and took that ocelot hat I've been wanting since I was, like, sixteen. It's so hot. Still smells a little like mothballs—she told me I could have it when she was dead! Oh, my God, I forgot to tell you! There's this consignment shop about thirty miles away. Everything in it is, like, two dollars. I'm not even kidding. I got the dress I'm wearing right now there. I wish you could see it. It's got real lace at the collar and only two rips, one at the waist, and well, the whole hem needs to be resewn but that's cool. I'll fix it tomorrow."

At the next table, I rummage through my briefcase in hopes of finding a few cyanide capsules or a firearm.

Vintage garments and accessories are fine—in moderation. Wear Grandma's old brooch on a cashmere cardigan. If you find a vintage tweed blazer that's in perfect condition and it fits, buy it. Pair it with jeans. Fabulous. What's not fabulous is walking down the street in 2011 looking as though you just time-traveled from 1942.

Vintage must fit. It must be in like-brand-new condition, and it must be made to look relevant through pairings with modern clothes.

Kooky!

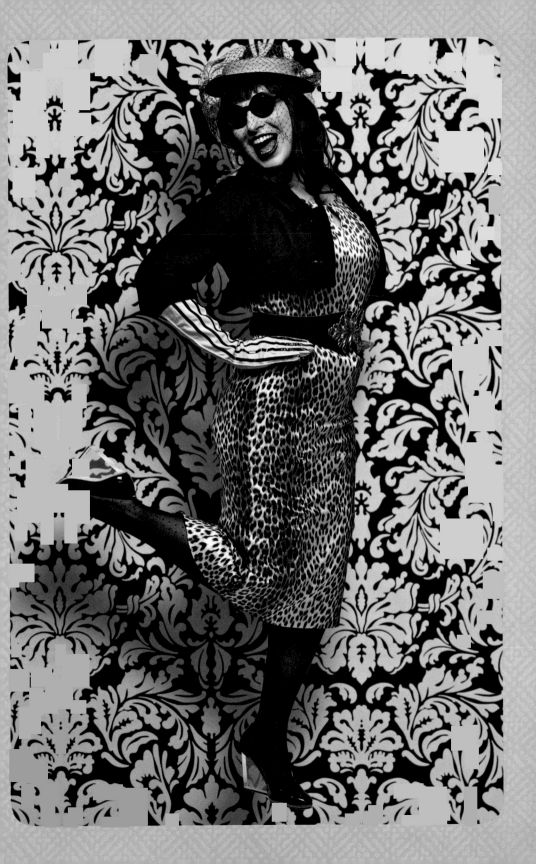

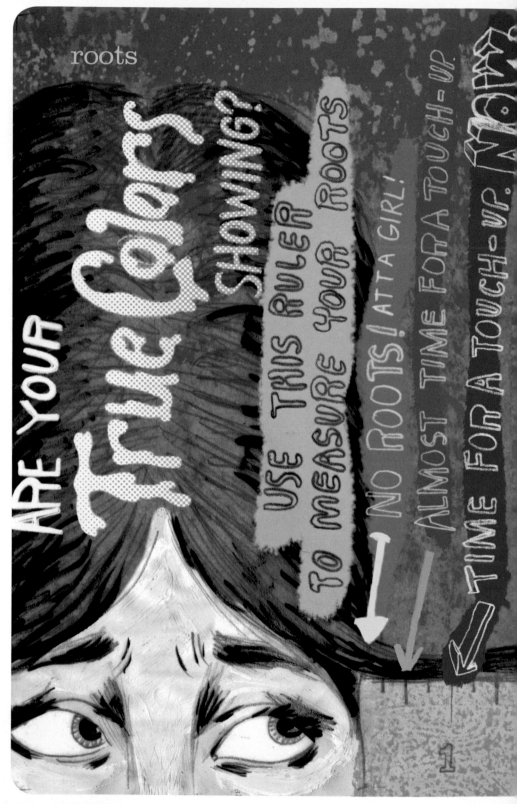

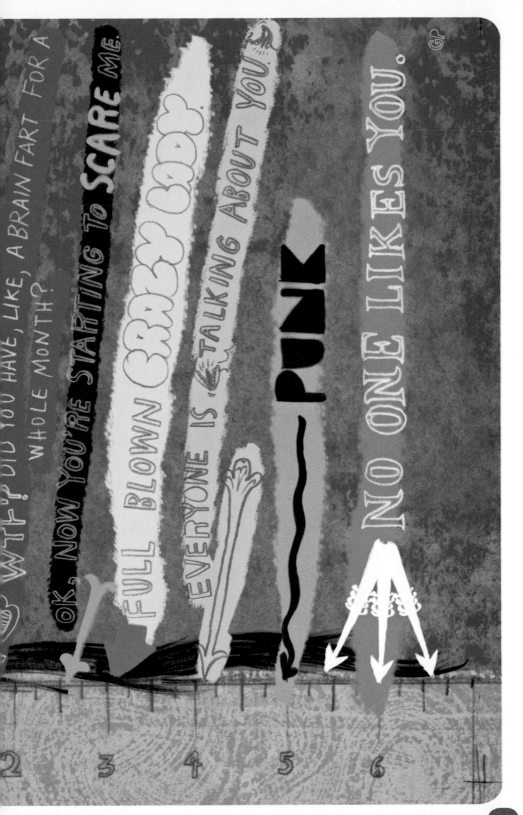

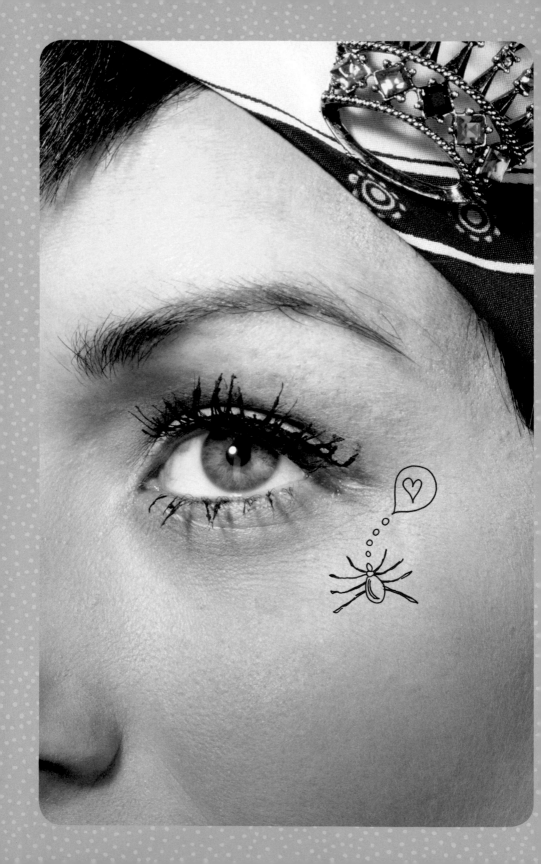

gloppy mascara

Maybe it's just me, but I always thought the point of mascara was to make your lashes look longer and thicker, thereby creating the illusion of bigger and prettier eyes. So, tell me then, why do I see at least one woman every day who appears to have applied asphalt to her lashes with a pitchfork? It's not cute. It makes me think you've just paved over a week's worth of eye boogers.

But as much as I'd like to blame *you* for this style sin, my pal Carmindy says I should blame your mascara wand. "The really big ones—and some of them are huge these days—tend to clump fastest," she says. Instead, choose a brand with a smaller brush so you can apply mascara to each individual lash, then build up to your desired thickness.

If you absolutely must have the fattest applicator on the market, Carmindy recommends keeping a folding lash comb handy so you can separate those suckers! And I agree, you two-bit Tammy Faye knockoff.

stirrup pants

Stirrup pants were big in the '80s. They recently made a comeback, which made me feel old. I can only imagine that it made you feel *ancient*.

If you want to wear stirrup pants because they're trendy, I couldn't care less. Have a freakin' ball with your fashionista friends, listening to Taylor Swift and drinking wine coolers. But if you've been wearing them without pause for the last few decades because you like their "ease and style," to quote a certain maternal grandmother of mine, you might want to rethink them as a wardrobe staple.

The legging is a decent alternative for some women. But keep in mind: anytime a pant narrows at the ankle, it must widen somewhere else. And that somewhere is your hips and thighs. If you don't mind widening those areas, knock yourself out.

If you want to wear leggings but you don't want your thighs to be the star of your show, wear them as you would tights or hose under a skirt or casual dress.

A note about yoga pants:

They are meant to be worn while performing ysga!!!...

If a downward-facing dog isn't in your immediate future, put on some real pants!

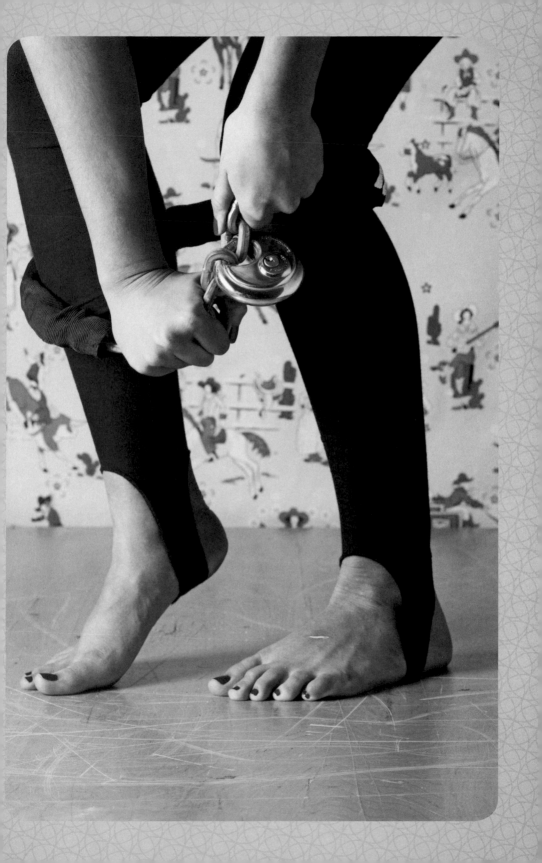

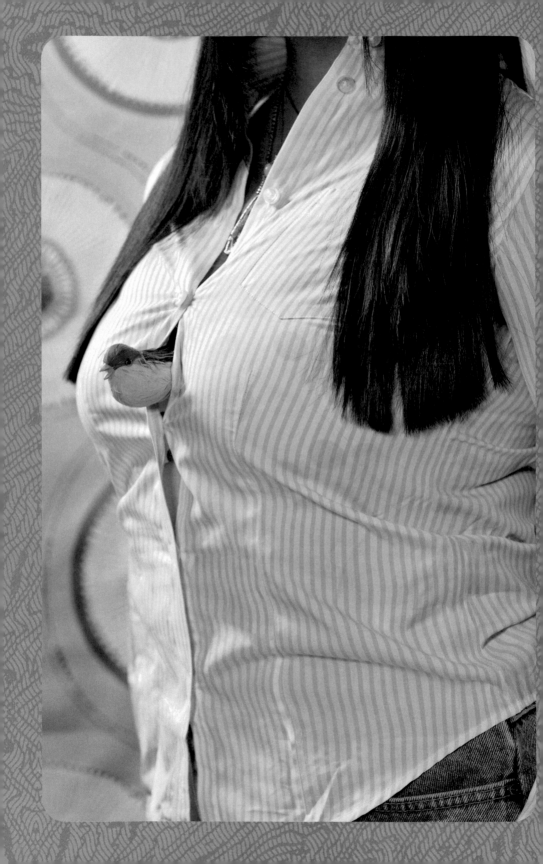

peekaboo, i see your boobies

Big ta-tas and button-front shirts go together about as well as peanut butter and mayonnaise. So women with ample bosoms often experience gaps between buttons when wearing them, which can often elicit gaping stares from nearby males. And really, who can blame them—it's distracting when the girls are struggling to bust out like two bear cubs wrestling in a bag.

The best way to prevent peekaboo action is to sew a little snap or two onto the placket of your shirt between buttons. They cost about a quarter and are an easy do-it-yourself fix. If snaps don't hold, try a hook-and-eye fastener. And if that doesn't work (or looks ridiculous because it's pulling so much), it means you are wearing a shirt that is too small. You must go up a size and tailor down. I know this seems like a lot of work and I probably sound like a broken record, but tailoring is something you have to get used to doing.

In the case of a woman with a large bust and a small waist, you must buy a shirt that fits comfortably across your girls. It may billow in the wind around your midsection, but that can be fixed with a few expertly sewn darts. Just do it and you'll have a button-front shirt that fits you perfectly and, more important, you can stop complaining about how nothing ever fits!

peep!

tiny logo bags

"You are not going to believe this, but my parents bought me, like, a new Coach bag for no reason at all!!! OMG, it's so cute!!! It's got all these Cs on it that stand for Coach, and I can fit, like, my cell phone and a tube of lip gloss and the keys to my dad's 2003 Acura in it. People are gonna totally think I'm rich. When I'm older, like twenty, and married and stuff, I'm gonna tell my husband that if he wants to have sex with me, he's gonna have to buy me a full-size Coach bag. I'm gonna be such a bitch like that. So, like, what shift are you working today? The four to twelve? Gross. I hate working that shift because all those snotty community college kids come in after school wanting fries, and I'm like, 'If you want to sit in a booth, you have to spend at least ten dollars.' And they're like, whatever, and I'm like, 'Here's your menu, smarty-pants. Your waitress will be right with you.'"

Nobody will think you're rich and famous if you carry around the smallest logo-covered bag the company makes and wear it with a velour tracksuit and flip-flops. It's like putting a Rolls-Royce hood ornament on your crappy Dodge Dart. Instead of looking like a wannabe, you might want to try looking like the best version of yourself. Try spending the same amount of money on a bag that doesn't rely on initials for its personality.

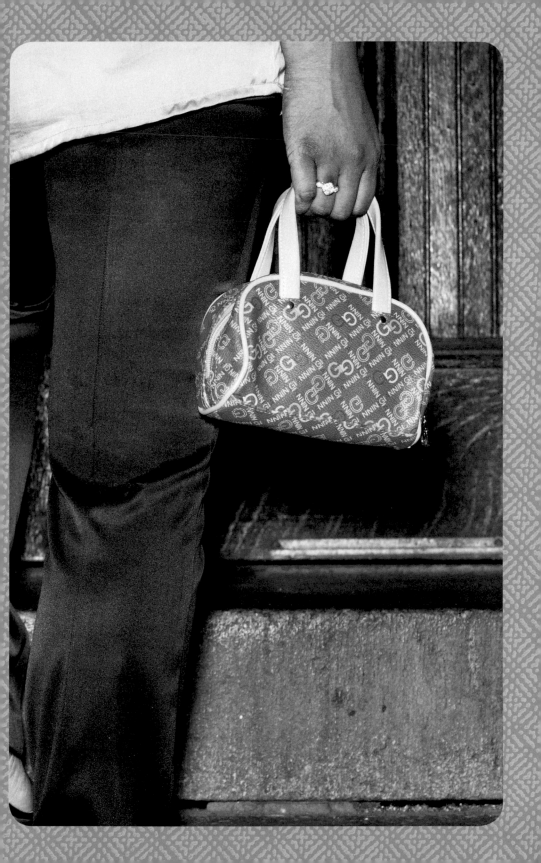

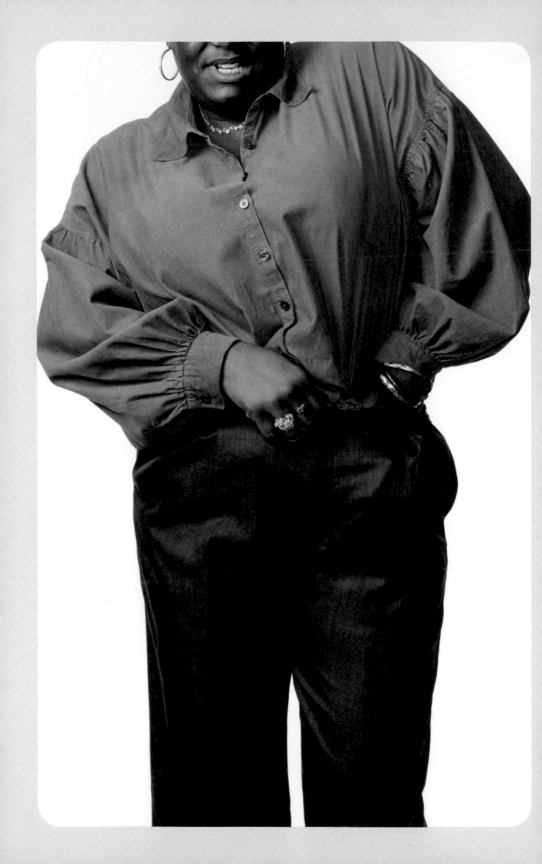

Stop stuffin'!

tucking

For the most part, both men and women would prefer a small waist to a larger one. That's why I have a job. I trick other people into thinking you have a smaller waist than you actually do.

Anytime you tuck your shirt into your pants (or skirt), you create a focal point. And that focal point is your waist. If your waist is small—no problems. But if your waist is thick, you've just turned your tummy into a focal point. Uh-oh.

You can counteract the effects of a tucked-in shirt by wearing a jacket. A jacket will pull the focus away from the tummy and redistribute it to the shoulder, lapel, and sleeve. If you've got a tummy and you don't want to wear a jacket, wear your tops untucked. *But* you can't do this with any old oversize top. You need a top that floats away from the tummy *and* keeps the leg line as long as possible.

visible pin jobs

Oh, the wonders of the safety pin. You can use them to keep a baby's cloth diaper closed or to scratch SKANK ever so lightly on the front door of the bitch who tried to steal your man— not so big that everyone can see it, just her, when she puts the key in the lock. But despite their infinite utility, safety pins should not be worn in lieu of seeing a tailor.

If your pants don't fit in the waist, don't pin them—take them to a tailor and have them taken in. If your pants are too long, don't pin them up—take them to a tailor and have them hemmed. If you have a rip in your jacket, don't pin it closed— take it to a tailor and have it repaired. I hope you're getting my drift, because if I had to make my point any simpler, it would be a cave painting.

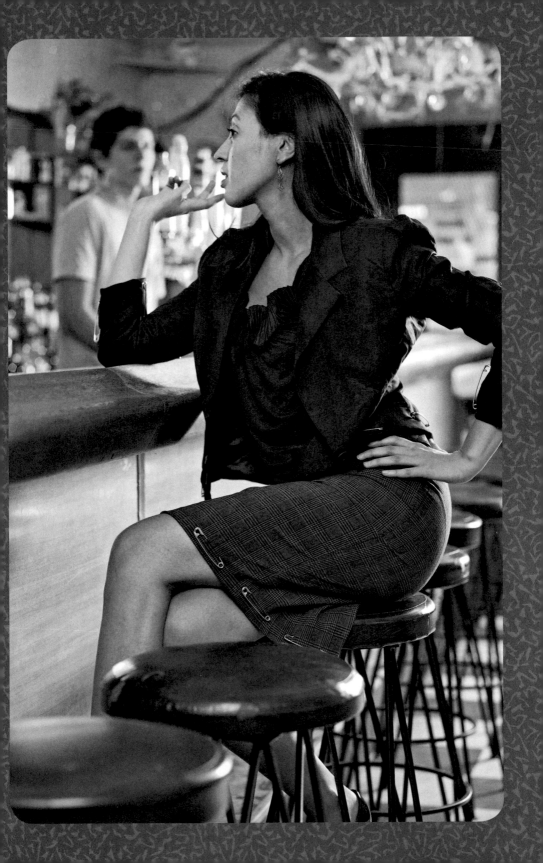

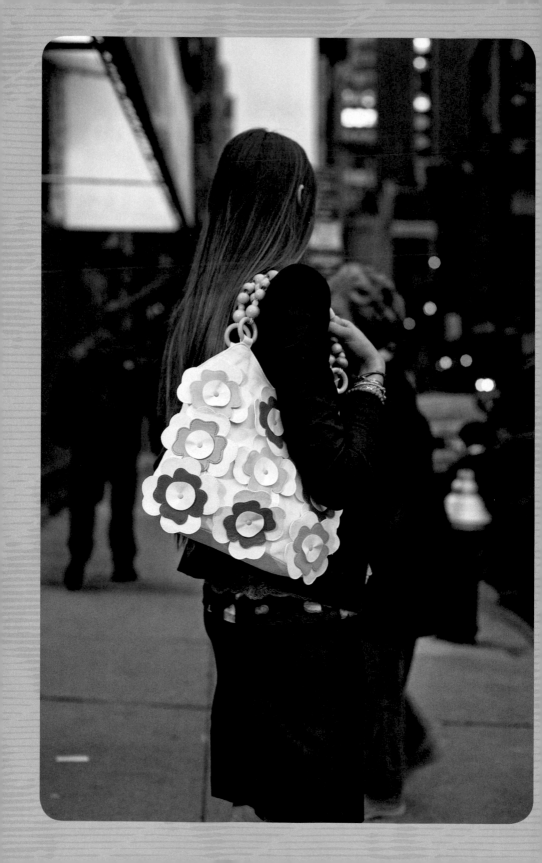

novelty bags

Answer: E. All of the above do not belong—anywhere on this planet.

Your bag tells the world of your status, so you should carry any of the above bags if your status falls somewhere between "circus freak" and "huge doofus."

Yes, bags are certainly a great way to add interest to an outfit. But don't rely on silly accessories to make people think you're interesting! (See Kooky Embroidery, page 188.) Use accessories to make yourself look current.

One of the best secrets of getting more mileage out of your wardrobe budget is to keep your clothes classic but sport a modern bag and shoe. Even a simple pair of herringbone trousers and a cashmere sweater can look super-relevant when worn with the bag of the moment, whether it's woven leather or patent or zippered or grommeted or whatever. Trust me on this one. And all the rest.

the boca sandal

Usually when I give a speech, I'll open up the floor to questions from the audience for fifteen minutes or so. This is always a little dangerous, because a lot of people in America are nuts. Not just a little kooky—but bat-shit crazy. But I like to live life on the edge. For example, once during a seminar I was hosting in front of a thousand or so retirees, a lady stood up and said, "I'm from Boca." (I knew exactly where this was going.) "Stop making fun of our city!" I asked her if she was carrying any concealed weapons. She said no, so I told her to lighten up and get a life. She got all huffy and frowned at me really intensely. But it didn't bother me, because I'm tough.

Yes, from time to time, when I see a woman in a white low square-heeled sandal, I will say, "Where'd you buy that shoe? Boca?" But that's only because most women who own that kind of shoe live in Boca. That's not making fun of a city, in my opinion. It's like when I see a guy with a Nissan Altima that has tinted windows and Jersey plates, I will say, "Where'd you get that car? Jersey?"

It's the same thing.

A flat strappy sandal is better than a white sandal with a low square heel. That's all I'm saying.

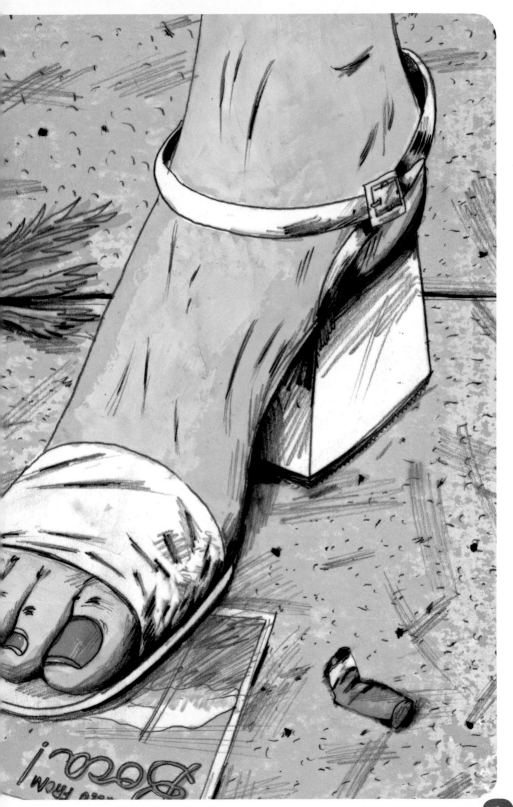

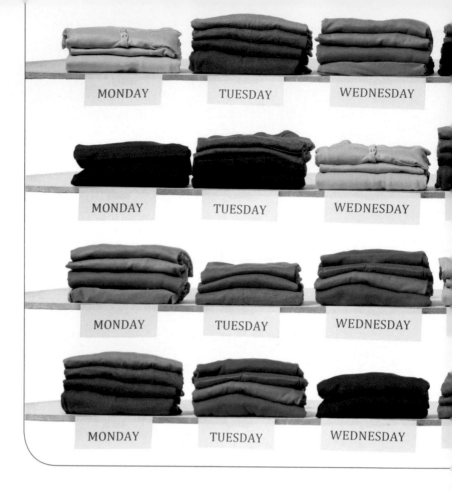

MONDAY   TUESDAY   WEDNESDAY

MONDAY   TUESDAY   WEDNESDAY

MONDAY   TUESDAY   WEDNESDAY

MONDAY   TUESDAY   WEDNESDAY

all solids all the time

Let's say you had a friend named Fran, and you and Fran enjoy going to nice restaurants. But every time you go out to dinner with Fran, she orders a salad. That's it. Every single time.

You go to Maine and order lobster; she has a salad. You go to Montana and have a steak; she has salad. You go to New Orleans and have gumbo; she has a salad. That's all. Salad, salad, salad.

You ask Fran, "Why don't you try something else for a change?" And she says, "Why? I like salad. Is there something wrong with salad?"

You say, "Of course there's nothing *wrong* with salad. But it's a big world out there, Fran, and I worry that you're missing out on some of it." After you say that, Fran goes berserk! She throws her salad at you and storms out of the restaurant. Everyone in the place thinks you've had a lover's quarrel, but you know better. You could never love someone like Fran. Then the waiter gives you the bill and motions to his own

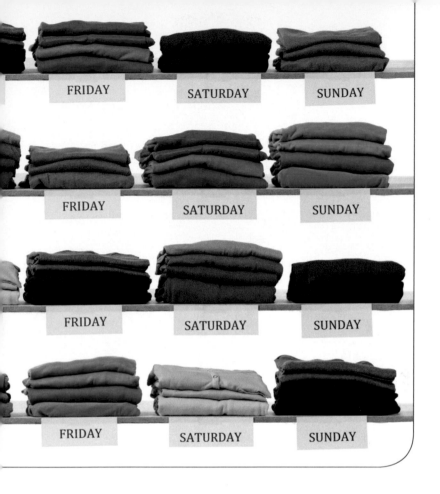

FRIDAY   SATURDAY   SUNDAY

FRIDAY   SATURDAY   SUNDAY

FRIDAY   SATURDAY   SUNDAY

FRIDAY   SATURDAY   SUNDAY

cheek. He's trying to tell you there's a little piece of carrot stuck to your face.

Well, solids are like salad. They're good, but too much of them make you a big ole bore.

Four ingredients make an outfit interesting:

Color!
Texture!
Pattern!
Shine!

You can add all four if you want. For example, a glen plaid trouser (pattern) worn with a violet blouse (color) and crocodile pumps (texture) and a gold multichain necklace (shine). Piece of cake.

Or you could do just two. A boldy printed dress (pattern) might just need a metallic shoe (shine).

And that's what I call salad dressing.

OH NO SHE DIDN'T

pubescent style

To determine whether you're too old to shop in the juniors department of your favorite department store or to wear brands that rhyme with Blabercrombie & Flitch, Kollister, and Shmamerican Beagle, take the quiz below!

Check each one that applies.

- Did you experience your first menstruation ten or more years ago?
- Can you legally order and consume a Long Island Iced Tea on Long Island?
- Have you ever seen an episode of *The Facts of Life* on prime-time network television?
- Speaking of TV, when you were a kid, did you have to get off the couch to change the channels?
- Do you remember when Bret Michaels used to be cool?
- Have you ever been called ma'am?

SCORING

One or more check marks:

You're too damn old to be dressing like a teenager!

Clothes sold in the juniors department are usually of lesser quality because teenagers are buying them, and nobody expects a teen to wear anything for more than a season. ("OMG, that's so eleventh grade.") Grown women who want to be known for having "style" should be focusing on quality first and foremost.

Juniors clothes are also designed for teen bodies, which are different from grown women's bodies, so the fit on an adult will never be quite right. And without good fit, you've got nothing. Also, juniors clothes are very heavily trend oriented in a teen kind of way. Let your kids look like kids. You've had your chance. Move on.

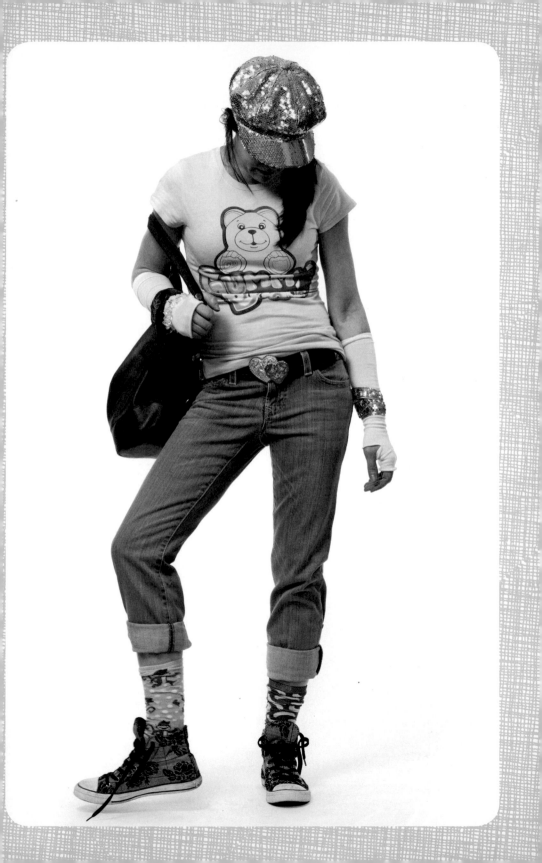

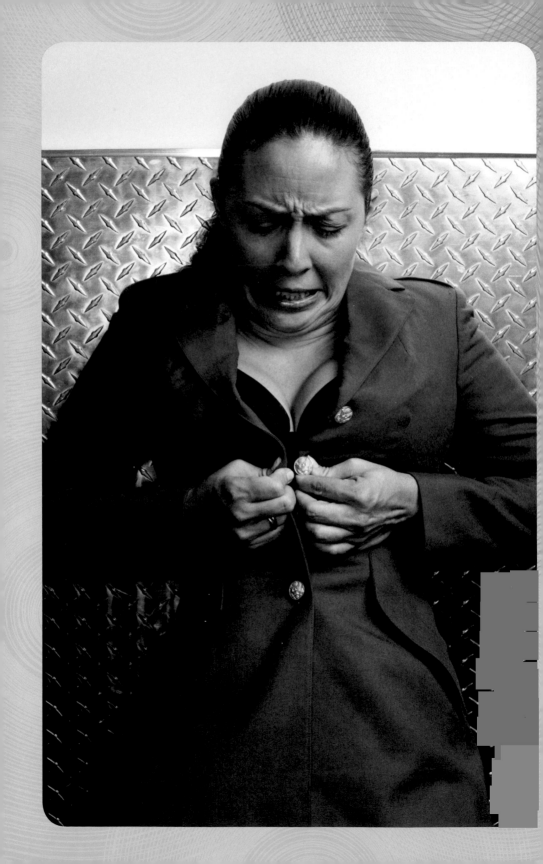

jackets that don't button

What's my mantra? "If you don't have fit, you don't have style. End of story." So . . . logically speaking, if a jacket doesn't close, it doesn't fit. And if it doesn't fit, you don't have style.

Sure, you can tell yourself that you're never going to wear it closed so it doesn't matter, but in psychological circles that's called *rationalization*. Other examples of rationalization include:

"The ice cream will go bad if I don't eat it."
"It's the cashier's fault for giving me an extra twenty."
"It's Vegas! And I brought antibiotics."

It's gotta close, babe. That's the whole purpose of a jacket. And I strongly believe that wearing a jacket that you can't close is psychological torture because you'll be reminding yourself all day *I'm too big for this jacket*. Please go up one size. And if the next size up is too big, tailor it down. Jackets are too important a wardrobe staple to settle for less than a perfect fit.

the little nubbin in the boat

Sometimes when a woman is wearing pants that are too tight in the thigh, too loose in the waist, and too high in the rise, she'll get a little nubbin in the crotch of her pants. Nobody will ever tell a woman she has great style if it appears she has a wiener.

I'll be honest with you, if you currently own pants that give you the junk-in-the-front look, they probably can't be fixed because the main culprit here is the tightness in the thigh, which is causing the pants to bunch up in the crotch. You need to either go up a size or look for pants that have a looser cut on the leg. If you go up a size to accommodate your thighs and the pants are now too big in the waist, what are you gonna do? Yes, that's right; you're going to have them taken in at the waist. You're getting good at this. (See Gap in the Back, page 84.)

Crotch watch!

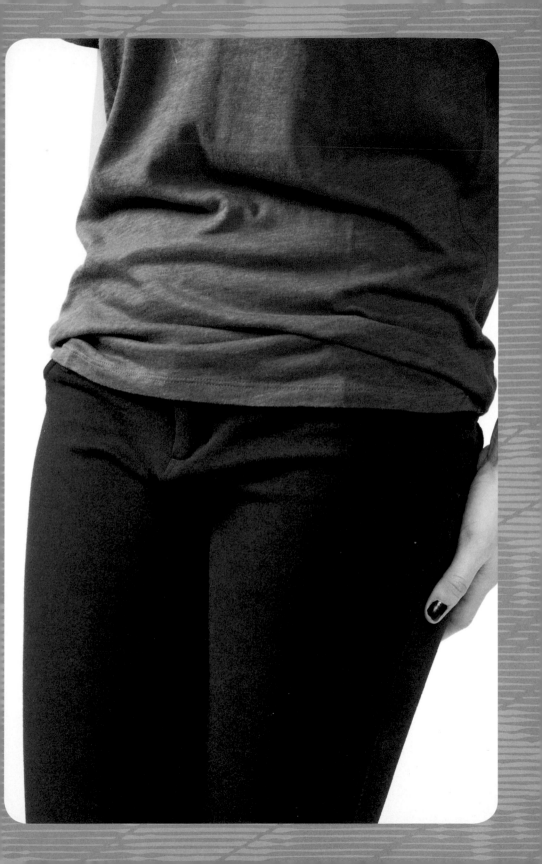

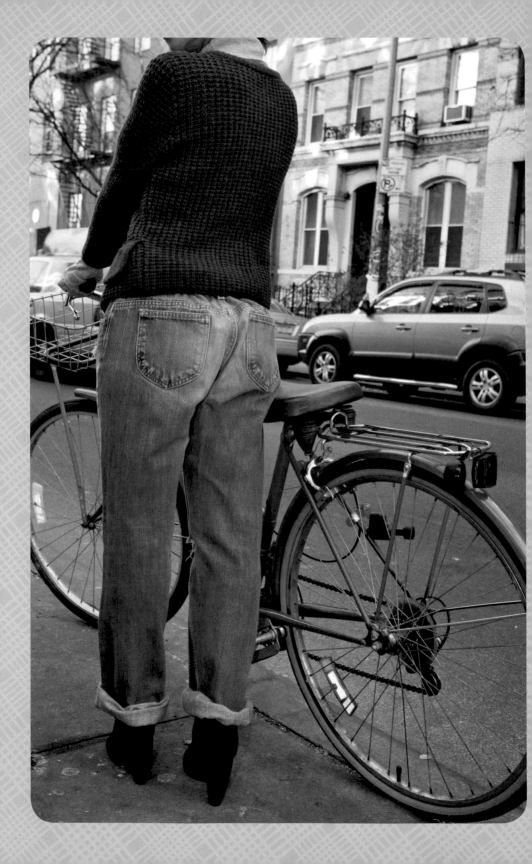

baggy butt

What I like about clothes most of all is they're the great equalizers—you don't have to have a fantastic body to have fantastic style. You might have boobs down to your knees and an ass with more wrinkles than a Shar-Pei—but *nobody else has to know about it* (except, of course, your spouse, which is why I always recommend having some piece of dirt on your significant other in case he or she starts mouthing off). So, there is no reason to be walking around in clothes that make your ass look anything less than fabulous.

Yes, it's true, if you don't have much of a butt, it is difficult to find pants that fit well off the rack. If this is the case and you have a small frame, I recommend wearing pants that fit very close to the body, such as a skinny jean or a legging. Flap pockets or other back-pocket detailing can help add a little more oomph to your ass too. Or you can do what I recommend for women with medium or larger frames who don't have much tush: Buy pants with the best fit you can find, that are comfortable at the waist and drape nicely on the leg. Then ask your tailor to take them in through the seat. Just so you know, while she's doing the fitting, she will be all up in your junk! She'll probably be just as uncomfortable with the whole process as you are, and afterward you can share a cigarette.

matching jewelry

I can kind of understand buying a pair of matching earrings and a necklace that come in one blue velvet box. But I don't quite get why a woman would wear them together. When your earrings match your necklace, it looks like you're wearing a "set," and a "set" doesn't say you have style. It says you don't have a mind of your own. Unless you're a Stepford wife, this is not how style works anymore. (See Matchy-Matchy Outfits, page 70.)

I was at a press conference recently, and I was talking to a reporter who had obviously put a lot of effort into her outfit. (I think she was trying to impress me, as people are inclined to do because I'm fabulous and judgmental.) Every item of clothing fit her, and overall her outfit was quite flattering. But around her neck she wore an opal pendant on a thin gold chain, and on each ear she wore matching opal pendants. It was so distracting! I kept looking from one ear to the other ear to her décolletage, back to one ear, then back down again, then up to one ear. The whole experience gave me a migraine.

If you have a favorite necklace, that's great. Wear it. Show it off. Don't distract from it by wearing its twin sisters on your ears. When accessorizing, you must decide which element will be the star of the show, the necklace or the earrings. It can't be both. Bold earrings? Go for a smaller or thinner necklace. Big necklace? Go with smaller studs or drops. Sometimes you can wear a bold necklace and bold earrings, but that's mostly for an evening or very formal event. Still, they should "go," but not "match" exactly.

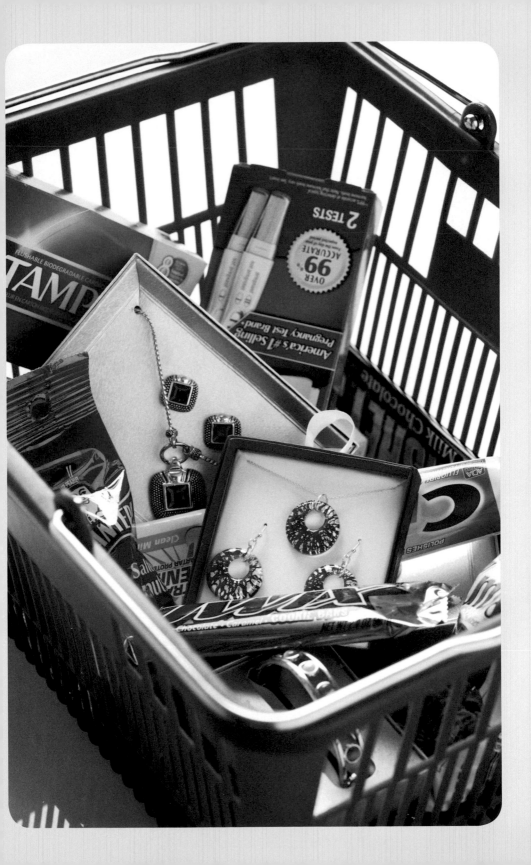

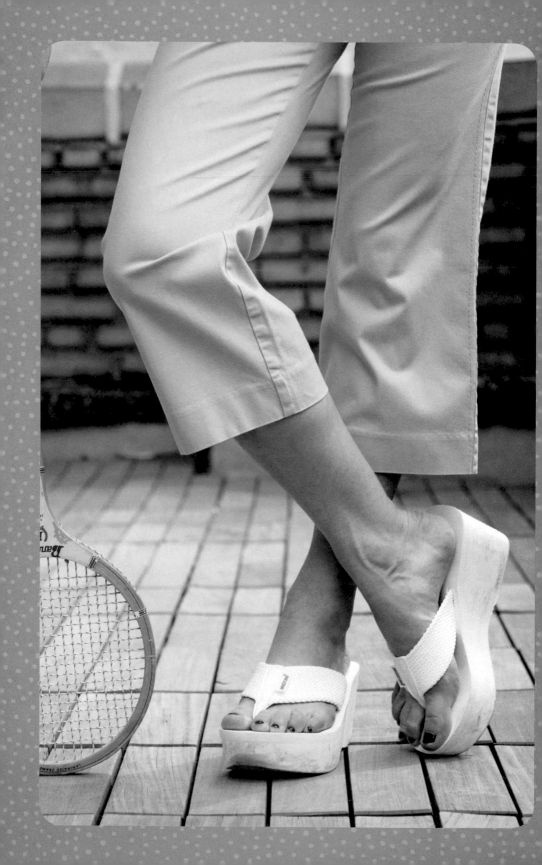

platform flip-flops

LADY AT MALL: (*Interrupting a conversation between my sister and me.*) I know you. You're that guy from that show. I watch that show all the time.

ME: You're wearing platform flip-flops.

LADY AT MALL: They're my daughter's.

ME: Some shoes should not be shared.

LADY AT MALL: You don't like them?

ME: Are you serious?

LADY AT MALL: They make me taller.

ME: So you wear them to get things off high shelves?

LADY AT MALL: Well, not really.

ME: You'd be better off carrying around a step stool. Then I might look at you and think: *That's a smart lady who knows she's short. She has places to go and things on high shelves to buy.* But now I look at you and think: *That's a short lady with bad footwear.*

LADY AT MALL: I thought you'd be nicer.

ME: I'm nice to people who don't wear platform flip-flops and don't interrupt me. Maybe you could be one of those people in the future.

LADY AT MALL: (*Leaving.*) Fuck off.

SISTER: Remember when they had Orange Julius at this mall?

ME: Those were the days, Sis. Yes, those were the days.

There is NO good reason for wearing a platform flip-flop. None. Zero. And if you're gonna interrupt me and ask, "Aren't you what's his name?" you had better prepare yourself to get read!

pilling

There are good pills and there are bad pills. For example, Xanax are good pills. Very good pills. The little dingleberries attached to your cashmere sweater, bad pills. These bad little pills are caused by friction, so they're usually located under the arms or at the sides of your bust.

I had a favorite sweater that pilled on the back because my Jack Spade messenger bag was rubbing against it. I was so mad at that Jack. Not just because of the pilling, but because I hated that show *Just Shoot Me!* starring David Spade. (They're related.)

To remove the pills, you can buy a little pill shaver and shave or pluck the suckers off before wearing. That's a lot of work for some of you, I know. Better is to prevent the pills from forming in the first place. Higher-quality wool and cashmere don't pill as much because the expensive stuff is made of longer fibers and pills are little balls that form from the smaller strands.

If higher-quality cashmere does pill, return it. I've brought sweaters back to stores after one wearing for unreasonable pillage. They always take it back, probably because they know I'll make a scene. Still, you should do the same. Also avoid carrying your bag up against your favorite sweater.

Sometimes a sweater is so pilled that it must be put down. Don't feel bad; the goat or sheep that it came from might still be alive on a beautiful farm somewhere, unless someone ate it.

A Xanax Haiku
by Clinton Kelly
You take the edge off
Fewer calories than wine
Generic's nice too

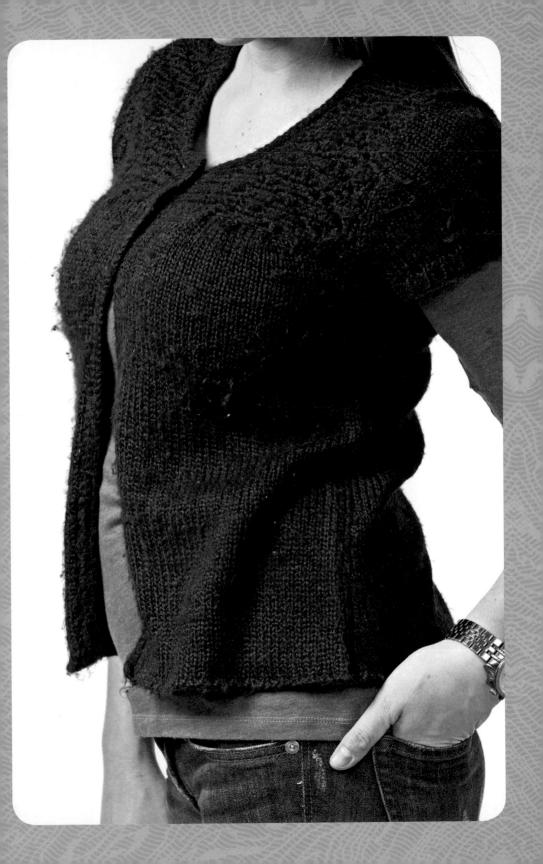

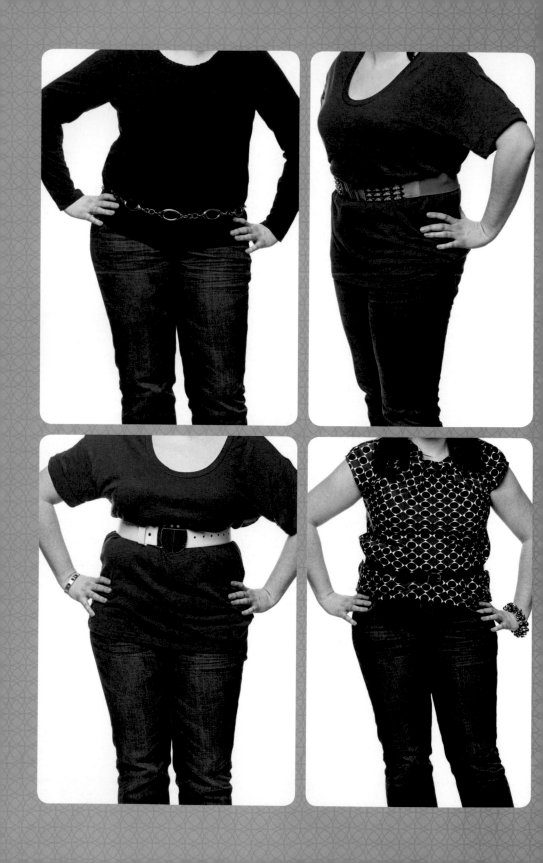

misguided belts

Belts bring attention to your midsection and define your waist. This is a good thing, sometimes. The waist is an incredibly important component of the hourglass shape, the essence of the female silhouette. So, if you have a narrow waist, belt it. But a woman's natural waist isn't always her smallest part, in which case it doesn't work to her advantage to direct attention toward it.

If you have a tummy, never put a belt right across the widest part of it, and definitely don't put the belt below the tummy. Yikes. You'll look like John Goodman.

Instead, try belting a blouse or a dress slightly higher than your natural waist. Nine times out of ten a woman's smallest part is under the bust, approximately mid-rib cage. This is your smallest part, so make a focal point of it, diverting attention away from your widest part.

A few more notes on belts. If you have a large frame, don't wear a skinny belt. It will look disproportionately thin, making you appear bigger. And a belt should feel snug but not tight; no flesh overflow.

bad posture

Your mother was right when she told you not to chase your diet pills with a rum and Tab. Oh, wait, that was my mother. Your mother was right when she told you to stand up straight.

Bad posture makes your boobs look droopy and your tummy pouchy. Plus, it makes other people think you're awkward and uncomfortable in your own skin. Don't ruin a perfectly cute ensemble by contorting yourself into a question mark.

When standing or sitting, think about pulling your shoulder blades back toward each other and down, and keep your core muscles slightly tightened. This is where all those Pilates DVDs you bought off that infomercial should pay off. Mine are still in the box. That was money well spent. Yep.

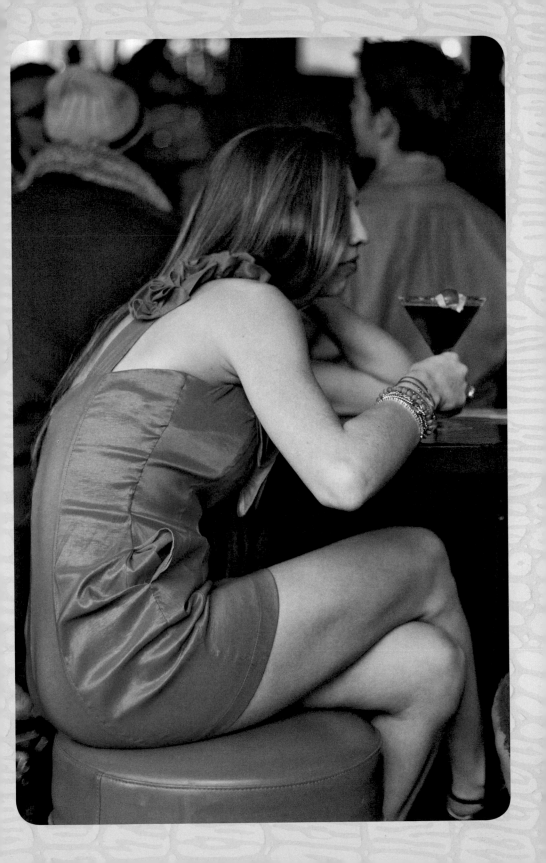

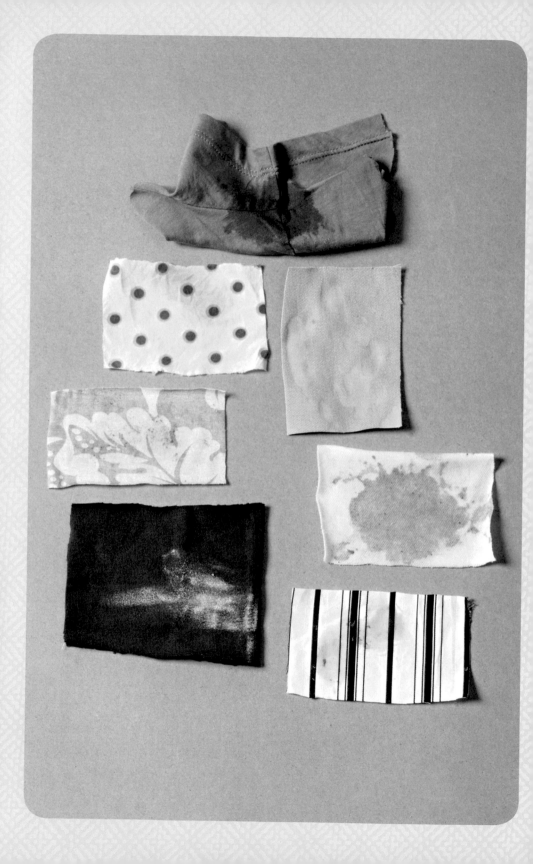

stains

All good things must come to an end. Like Nick Nolte's career.

If you cannot remove a stain, the garment is unwearable, dead, *finito*. Just let it go and say good-bye. Stains make you look dirty. Not "I enjoy having my toes sucked" dirty, more like "I haven't cleaned my toilet in three months" dirty. And that's nasty.

The next time you have the urge to hang onto a stained shirt you can wear while you paint the bathroom, ask yourself this: "When was the last time I actually engaged in any home improvement project?" If the answer is more than six months ago, stop kidding yourself. You're just not the type of woman who enjoys manual labor. You don't need a "work shirt." You need a daiquiri and a pedicure.

If you're the kind of woman who replaces grout for fun and does her own landscaping, I will allow you a maximum of two stained garments in your wardrobe, which will be stored in the garage—not your bedroom closet. That's right. Your closet should be your sanctuary of fabulousness. Don't clog it up with crap.

The best way to avoid stains is to prevent them from setting in the first place, so use a pretreatment product like _____*. Then launder your garment in cold water. If the stain doesn't lift, don't put the garment in the dryer; it could set the stain permanently. Instead, soak it in ____* and repeat until the stain lifts.

*Please note, any clothing care products that would like to sponsor this page in future printings, call my people.

kooky embroidery

I'm amazed sometimes that certain garments are ever sold. There are *a lot* of steps involved in getting clothing into stores, and—it seems—*a lot* of lapses in judgment in allowing this stuff to see the light of day. First someone has to design the garment. Then a retail buyer places an order for 10,000 of them. Then another group of people produces them. Then another group of people dresses mannequins and stocks store shelves. Then more people ring them up at cash registers.

So how does it happen that nobody along that chain of command doesn't scream at the top of her lungs, *"The world does not need ten thousand denim shirts embroidered with little bunny rabbits and carrots!"*

Personally, I think someone should be punished. And I think it should be the designer who conceived the notion in the first place. I mean, you can't buy cold medicine in this country anymore without showing ID because someone might use it in a meth lab. Yet people can create this wearable garbage. They shouldn't be allowed to purchase the thread without a taste license.

You might think that little leprechauns or flamingos or panda bears or umbrella-toting ducks are cute, but they're not. They're silly, and when you wear them you look silly. I've had women tell me, "But people smile when they see my teddy bear shirt!" And to that I say, "They're smiling because that's what you do around people who are mentally challenged."

Don't turn yourself into a joke. If you want to make people happy, develop a sense of humor or do nice things or get a job as a goddamn clown.

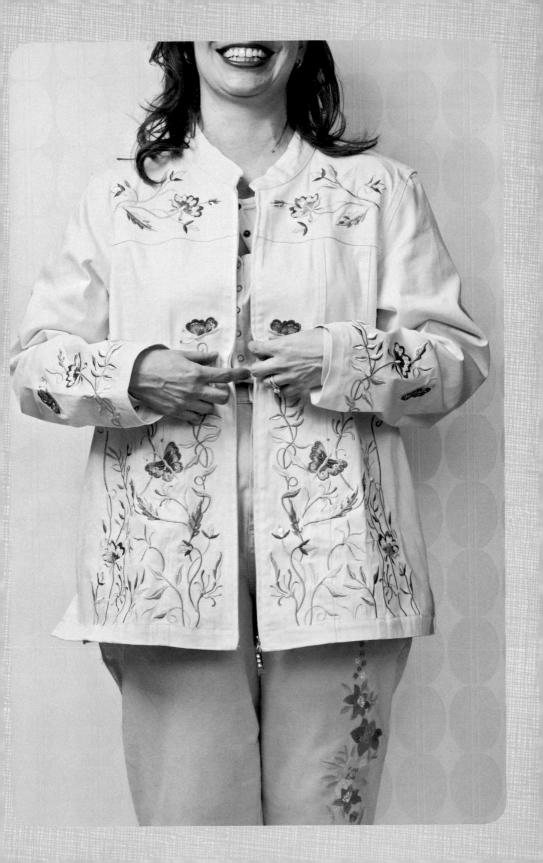

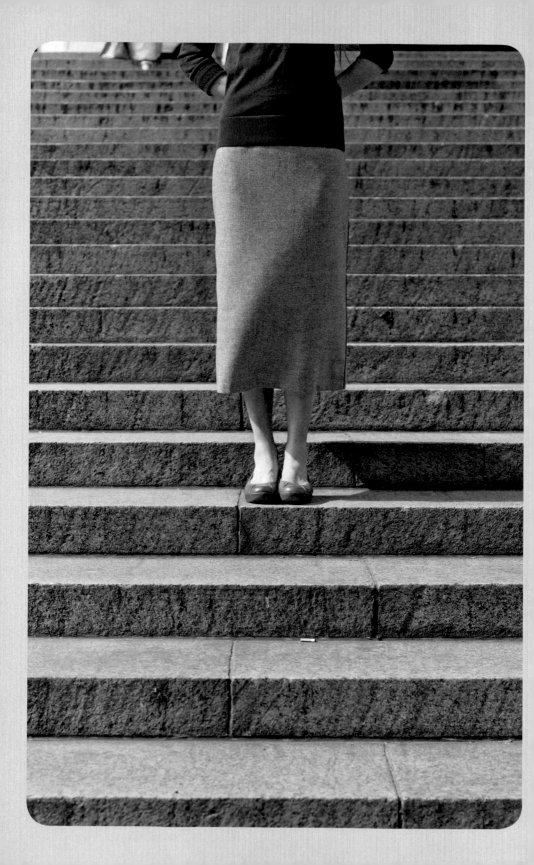

calf-length skirts

If you want to give other people the impression that you're a member of a religious cult, go get yourself a calf-length straight skirt. Yuck. I can't stand 'em!

In general, pencil skirts, A-line skirts, and straight skirts look best when the hem hits somewhere around the knee. For the best proportion, petite women should aim for the top of the kneecap. On taller women, skirts that reach the bottom of the knee usually work well. That's just a general rule of thumb, however. Skirt length and proportion depend not just on a woman's height but also the size of her frame, how big her bust is in comparison to her hips, and what height heel she's wearing. And sometimes determining ideal length is more art than science. So, when in doubt, aim for the knee.

Occasionally, a woman will tell me she hates her kneecaps. Personally, I think life is too short to feel such contempt for your patellae. But if your knees aren't the bee's knees, hem your skirts to the bottom of your 'cap—but not longer.

If you're choosing longer dresses because you don't like your legs, just wear pants. Honestly. A calf-length skirt isn't going to camouflage anything. You'd be better off with beautiful trousers and a fierce shoe.

That's my opinion. I'm stickin' to it. And please keep your pamphlets to yourself.

mini anything over "a certain age"

There will come a time in every woman's life when she will ask herself, "Am I too old to wear a skirt this short?" And the answer is yes—at least if you're talking about something that hits midthigh or higher. Here's why: You might have really amazing legs for your age, and are not afraid to show them off at a party. But I guarantee that they're not going to be as perfect as the gams on the twenty-two-year-old model attending the same event. She's going to walk into that room and everyone will be subconsciously comparing your legs to hers. And she wins—because she's twenty-freakin'-two!

The trick is to make sure that implicit rivalry never occurs. A woman over a certain age should give the impression that she is beautiful and feels no need whatsoever to compete with women half her age. The sexiest thing a woman can ever, ever have is confidence.

I love when I tell a woman she shouldn't wear a mini and she says, "But what about Tina Turner?" And I say, "Tina Turner is a performer. When you have ten thousand people paying to watch you sing 'Proud Mary,' you can wear a minidress too."

"But what about Demi Moore?" she might ask.

I reply, "Demi Moore is a movie star. You are a mom of three from Columbus, who works in pharmaceutical sales. And Demi Moore is married to a man barely out of puberty. *This* is your role model?"

Now, to address the pink elephant in the room, how old is "a certain age"? If you think I'm going to answer that, you are crazier than everyone says you are. It is up to a woman to decide that for herself, but if she decides it's sixty, she's about twenty years too late.

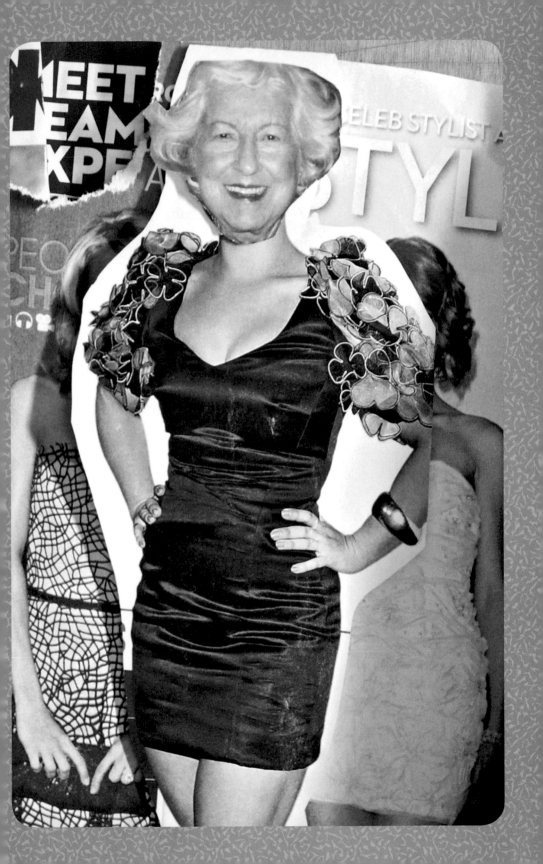

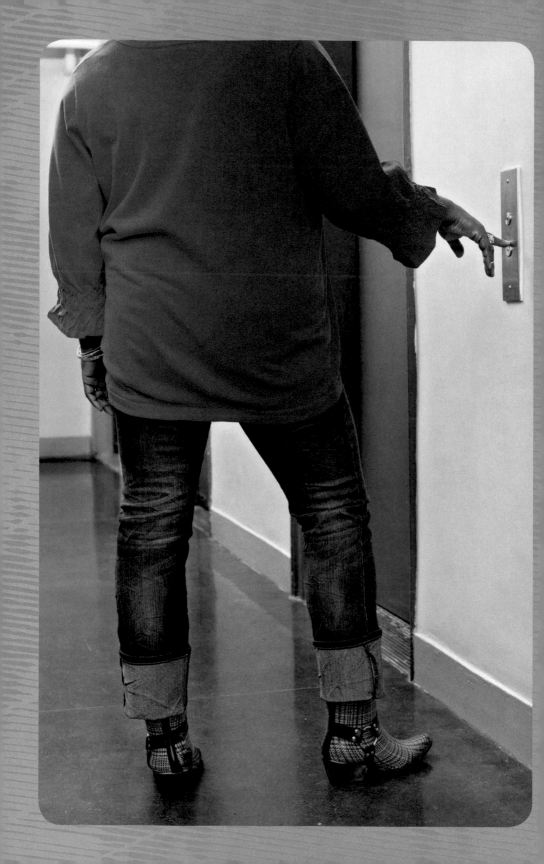

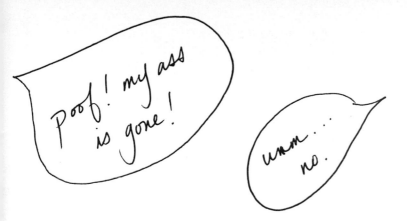

covering your ass with an invisibility cloak

Oh, wouldn't it be nice if there existed a magic blanket, which you could throw on top of a problem, and that problem would just disappear forever? Think of how great life would be! A stack of unpaid bills—*poof*—they never existed! Dog poop on your new silk rug—*poof*—gone, with no residual odor! Your lazy stepson—*poof*—Tyler who?

Unfortunately, this trick does not work when you cover your ass with a sweatshirt. Guess what, Mary, *we all know it's still there.*

The best way to camouflage your rear end is to use what I call the "divide and conquer" technique. Look for tops that hit at the widest part of the tush. I know that sounds counterintuitive, but it works. Think of it this way: if your tops are very short and hit above the butt, then everyone can see your entire butt and it becomes the primary focus of your rear view. If your tops are very long, your entire butt is covered, but your silhouette will look very wide and your leg line will look shorter. (Shorter legs mean you look shorter, and when you look shorter, you look wider.) *But,* if you cover the tush halfway, you bisect the butt, reducing its emphasis by half, and keep the leg line nice and long.

mall jewelry

Name any style icon, living or dead, and I can guarantee you with no degree of uncertainty that she did not buy her jewelry at a kiosk located within fifty feet of a Panda Express. I'm certainly not saying you can't find decent accessories at the mall. Of course you can, but little birthstone kid charms don't count as decent. Jewelry is a status indicator, and dinky jewelry always, always, always makes you look cheap, cheap, cheap. One of the best things about America is our ability to knock off expensive stuff really quickly (usually with the help of China, our semifriendly neighbor across the Pacific).

Keep in mind that a knockoff is not a fake (see Counterfeit Anything, page 20); a knockoff is something, ummm, heavily inspired by an original and is incredibly common in the fashion world. But to determine whether buying a knockoff is worthwhile, you have to know what's going on in the fashion world. So pick up one of those style magazines from time to time and see what kind of jewelry the It girls are wearing. An affordable facsimile will likely make its way to the mall before you can finish that egg roll.

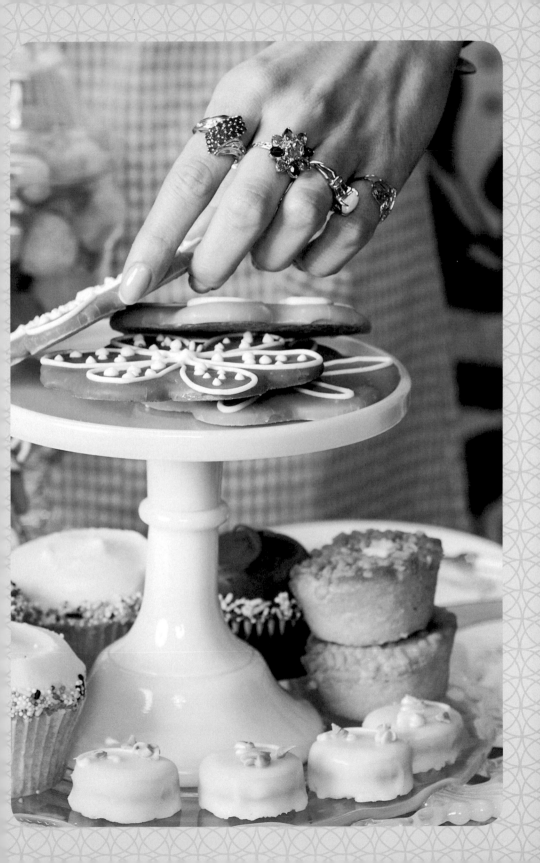

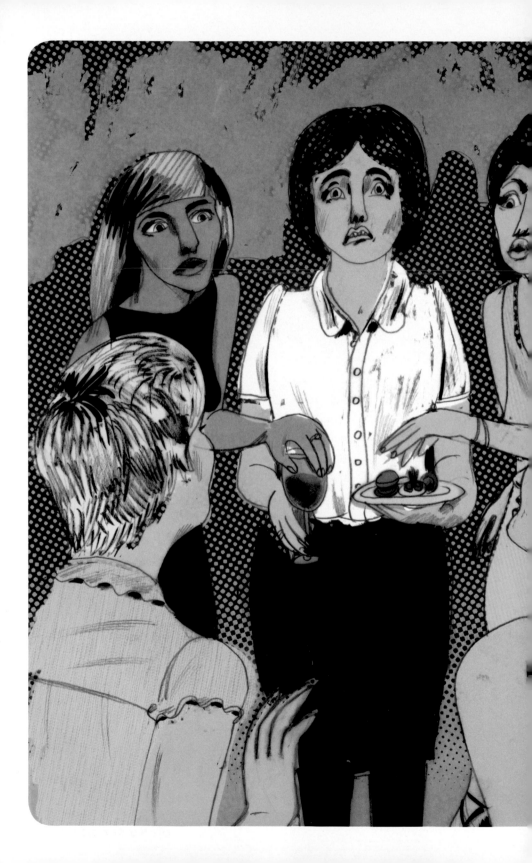

black pants and white shirts

I grew up on Long Island, which is famous for many things, mostly its beautiful beaches and overly confrontational people with heavy accents. It's also got more diners per capita than anyplace on Earth. *

* Don't quote me on that. I was too lazy to look it up, but it seemed true.

Although, New Jersey might have it beat. Same difference, really.

And what do diner waitresses wear? Black pants and a white shirt, usually with a Manhattan clam chowder stain on the sleeve. If it's a fancy diner, they might wear a black vest. This allows the owner to charge $15.99 for an open-face turkey sandwich worth $5.99.

It's not very chic to be mistaken for food service personnel. Not that there's anything wrong with working in a restaurant. I waited tables for eight years. Not the best career choice for someone with a superiority complex. I would give people disapproving looks for ordering a well-done filet mignon or for holding their knives incorrectly. I even told several rude customers not to "take that tone with me." It's always fun to see what kind of tip they leave you after that. A whopping 3 percent? Ouch, that hurts. By the way, I put Visine in your coffee. * * Have fun on the drive home.

* * Don't put Visine in anyone's food. It could kill them!

If you are going to wear black pants, do so with a neutral-colored or printed top. If you're going to wear a white blouse, do so with a printed skirt or patterned trousers. Or add a colored sweater.

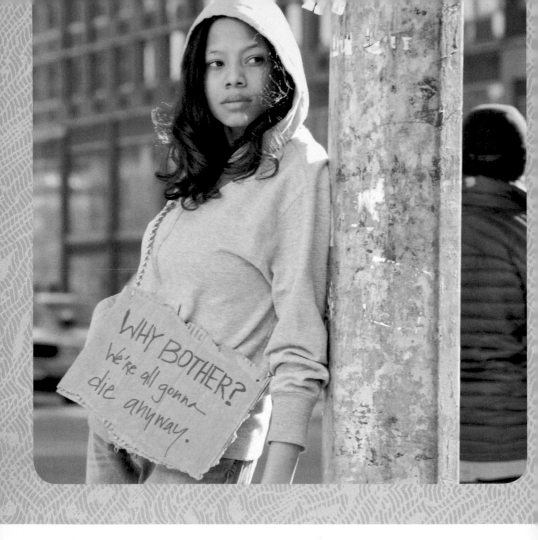

opting out

This is where I give my big speech about trends and why it's important to participate in them, to some extent, for as long as you want to remain relevant in society. If you'd prefer to be left alone on your ranch with your husband and his other wives, you can just skip this section.

Whatever you do, don't opt out of trends altogether. It makes people think that you don't matter, but I'm here to tell you that you *do* matter, and Clinton loves you. Unless you're a jerk, then I don't love you.

Many women tell me they think trends are for younger women, and the truth is, some trends *are* meant solely for younger women—up to roughly their early thirties—but not *all* trends. Any given season, there might be twenty trends that designers are serving up for the masses,